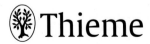

Pocket Atlas of Tongue Diagnosis

With Chinese therapy guidelines for acupuncture, herbs, and nutrition

Claus C. Schnorrenberger, M.D.
Professor and Director
German Research Institute of Chinese Medicine
Freiburg im Breisgau, Germany
Chairman of the Board of Directors
Lifu International College of Chinese Medicine
Basel, Switzerland

Beate Schnorrenberger
Naturopath and food chemist
Berlin, Germany

189 illustrations

Thieme
Stuttgart · New York

Library of Congress Cataloging-in-Publication Data

Schnorrenberger, Claus C., 1937 –
Pocket atlas of tongue diagnosis: with Chinese therapy guidelines for acupuncture, herbs, and nutrition / Claus C. Schnorrenberger, Beate Schnorrenberger.
p.; cm.
Includes bibliographical references and indexes.
ISBN 3-13-139831-0 (alk. paper) –
ISBN 1-58890-357-5 (alk. paper)
1. Tongue manifestations of general diseases – Atlases.
2. Medicine, Chinese – Atlases.
[DNLM:
1. Tongue – physiopathology – Atlases.
2. Tongue – physiopathology – Handbooks.
3. Acupuncture Therapy – Atlases.
4. Acupuncture Therapy – Handbooks.
5. Diagnosis, Differential – Atlases.
6. Diagnosis, Differential – Handbooks.
7. Medicine, Chinese Traditional – Atlases.
8. Medicine, Chinese Traditional – Handbooks.
9. Nutrition Therapy – Atlases.
10. Nutrition Therapy – Handbooks.
11. Oral Manifestations – Atlases.
12. Oral Manifestations – Handbooks.
13. Phytotherapy – Atlases.
14. Phytotherapy – Handbooks.
WI 17 S362p 2005]
I. Schnorrenberger, Beate. II. Title.

RC73.3.S37 2005
616.07'54 – dc22

2004026558

This book is an authorized and revised translation of the German edition published and copyrighted 2002 by Hippokrates Verlag, Stuttgart, Germany. Title of the German edition: Taschenatlas der Zungendiagnostik
Translated from the German edition by Claus C. Schnorrenberger, M.D.
e-mail: lifu@gmx.ch

© 2005 Georg Thieme Verlag,
Rüdigerstrasse 14, 70469 Stuttgart, Germany
http://www.thieme.de
Thieme New York, 333 Seventh Avenue, New York, NY 10001, USA
http://www.thieme.com

Cover design: Martina Berge, Erbach

Typesetting by OADF, 71155 Altdorf
www.oadf.de

Printed in Germany by Druckhaus Götz, Ludwigsburg

ISBN 3-13-139831-0 (GTV)
ISBN 1-58890-357-5 (TNY)   1 2 3 4 5

Important note: Medicine is an ever-changing science undergoing continual development. Research and clinical experience are continually expanding our knowledge, in particular our knowledge of proper treatment and drug therapy. Insofar as this book mentions any dosage or application, readers may rest assured that the authors, editors, and publishers have made every effort to ensure that such references are in accordance with **the state of knowledge at the time of production of the book**.

Nevertheless, this does not involve, imply, or express any guarantee or responsibility on the part of the publishers in respect to any dosage instructions and forms of applications stated in the book. **Every user is requested to examine carefully** the manufacturers' leaflets accompanying each drug and to check, if necessary in consultation with a physician or specialist, whether the dosage schedules mentioned therein or the contraindications stated by the manufacturers differ from the statements made in the present book. Such examination is particularly important with drugs that are either rarely used or have been newly released on the market. Every dosage schedule or every form of application used is entirely at the user's own risk and responsibility. The authors and publishers request every user to report to the publishers any discrepancies or inaccuracies noticed. If errors in this work are found after publication, errata will be posted at www.thieme.com on the product description page.

Some of the product names, patents, and registered designs referred to in this book are in fact registered trademarks or proprietary names even though specific reference to this fact is not always made in the text. Therefore, the appearance of a name without designation as proprietary is not to be construed as a representation by the publisher that it is in the public domain.

Preface

"Your eyes shall be your professors!"
—THEOPHRASTUS PARACELSUS (1493–1541)

J. W. Goethe, German writer, poet, and natural scientist of the 18th and early 19th century, once remarked: "The most difficult job is to recognize what is exposed in front of your eyes." What he meant was that you must know and understand the subject and its background thoroughly before you can explain it properly. Without this knowledge and understanding it is impossible to describe something accurately or even to see it at all. As far as tongue diagnosis is concerned this requires understanding human anatomy, physiology, and embryology, as well as Chinese medicine.

The human tongue undergoes constant change. It reflects every modification within the organism, as well as in the environment. We do, therefore, encourage the reader to inspect her or his tongue several times a day in order to well distinguish its body, its coating, its consistency, and the continuous changes involved. The mirror will each time reflect a slightly different picture and the tongue always reveals the actual phase of flow (or "equilibrium of flow") according to the prevailing individual syndrome, the *bian zheng*. The appropriate therapy should be applied in accordance with this. It is understood that the *bian zheng*, the differentiation of the individual syndrome, changes continuously, sometimes from hour to hour.

The procedure in Chinese diagnostics is the perennial differentiation between opposites. It is the vital medical application of the famous **Principle of Contradiction**, which in occidental thought goes back to Heraclitus, Parmenides, Plato, Aristotle, and Hegel, as well as to basic medical and diagnostic texts in the Chinese tradition (e. g., Chapter 49 of the *Ling-Shu Jing*). **Differentiation** based on **contradiction** is the correct rendering of the ideograph "*bian*," which is derived from a primitive ancient Chinese character showing two criminals impeaching each other. Thus, "*bian*" is the exact equivalent of Aristotle's *antiphasis*, namely contradiction, which he declared the basic principle of logic, analysis, and cognition in his book on metaphysics. Therefore, administering a typecast herbal prescription or a standard needle combination unthinkingly would be quite unprofessional.

The great compilations of classical prescription (*Shang Han Lun*, *Jin-Gui-Yao-Lüe*, Thousand Golden Prescriptions, etc.) give recommendations to the physician in order to suggest an appropriate creative therapy. Chinese physicians wrote them for this purpose some 2000 years ago. That is why the materia medica combinations listed in Chapters 5 to 8 have remained without standard quantification of their components. Quantification is up to the experienced physician according to the individual *bian zheng*. Moreover, quantification varies slightly between the Chinese and Western population and between people living in different climatic zones. Just copying stereotyped prescriptions and applying them to a sick person is as unprofessional a procedure as treating a diagnosis in the foreground instead of understanding the whole background (mind, organism, environment) of the individual human being involved.

An experienced Chinese doctor has to perform a comprehensive differentiating syndrome diagnosis (*bian zheng*) before his or her therapy, including inspection of the tongue and evaluation of pulses. Otherwise, the ensuing therapy would not be a genuine traditional Chinese one.

In conclusion, we would like to mention that the text of this atlas with its illustrations is based on a documentary film entitled *Zungendiagnose—Zentrum der Chinesischen Medizin* (Tongue diagnosis—The core of Chinese medicine) published in 1990 by the German Research Institute of Chinese Medicine (GRICMED), Freiburg im Breisgau/Germany.

Basel and Berlin,   The authors
November 2004

Contents

Foundations

Methodology of Tongue Diagnosis

Clinical Part

Appendix

1 Introduction and Preliminary Remarks

Overview of the Ten Chapters and the Appendices

- Chapter 2 contains a revision of the tongue's most important anatomical and physiological features.
- Chapter 3 explains the technique of tongue diagnosis.
- Chapter 4 presents a systematic classification of tongue structures based on more than 50 illustrations.
- Chapter 5 combines typical modifications of the body, the consistency, and the coating of the tongue with relevant therapeutic approaches (acupuncture, prescriptions, dietetics).
- Chapter 6 deals with typical changes of the tongue that are related to syndrome differentiation (*bian zheng*).
- Chapter 7 explains the course and development of some diseases, documented by illustrations.
- Chapter 8 shows the tongue photographs of 14 patients diagnosed with "headache (or migraine)" who required different individual treatment according to their different syndromes.
- Chapter 9 deals with modern research concerning tongue diagnosis.
- Albert Einstein's and a young chimpanzee's tongue inspired the authors to write the summary and outlook in Chapter 10.

The Appendix includes

1. Selected bibliographical references and figure sources,
2. The food groups according to the five elements,
3. The 21 groups of Chinese Materia Medica,
4. An alphabetical list of 370 medicinal herbs, minerals, and animal products,
5. Indexes of names and terms.

The Tongue Reflects all the Basic Phenomena of Chinese Medical Teachings

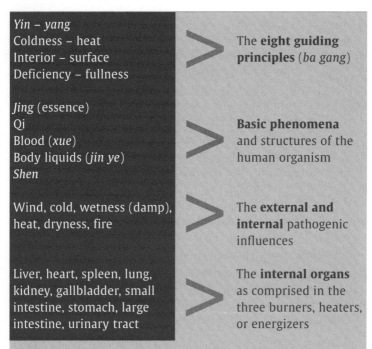

Yin – yang
Coldness – heat
Interior – surface
Deficiency – fullness

> The **eight guiding principles** (*ba gang*)

Jing (essence)
Qi
Blood (*xue*)
Body liquids (*jin ye*)
Shen

> **Basic phenomena** and structures of the human organism

Wind, cold, wetness (damp), heat, dryness, fire

> The **external and internal** pathogenic influences

Liver, heart, spleen, lung, kidney, gallbladder, small intestine, stomach, large intestine, urinary tract

> The **internal organs** as comprised in the three burners, heaters, or energizers

In addition, important pathological features of Chinese medicine
■ Blood blockage (xue yu), and
■ Phlegm or mucus (tan yin)
can be evaluated by analyzing the appearance of the tongue.

Documentary and Clinical Prerequisites

This atlas is the result of more than 30 years in medical practice. Research, photography, and documentation were performed at the German Research Institute of Chinese Medicine (GRICMED) in Freiburg im Breisgau/Germany. An initial series of tongue photographs was already taken between 1974 and 1976. The medical author, Dr. Claus Schnorrenberger, took numerous additional photographs during his clinical work in China (Shanghai and Hong Kong) and in the West (Freiburg and London). The nutritional recommendations including the survey of groups of food and nutriments were compiled by the co-author, Beate Schnorrenberger. They are based on many years of clinical experience in her own practice in Berlin.

Significance of the Tongue for the Human Individual and Mankind

The development of the tongue in the embryo reveals its close relationship with the origin of the human organism: the three germ layers of ectoderm, endoderm, and mesoderm (cf. p. 25). Thus, the tongue is an ontogenetic key organ for understanding the morphological and physiological intercommunication within the body. Moreover, the human tongue (Lat. *lingua*, Fr. *langue*, Germ. *Zunge*) is an essential element of human culture in general. Languages and intellectual conceptions, as well as the entirety of verbal terminology start with the tongue. This was taken into account quite early in the *Ling-Shu Jing* by associating the tongue with the heart and, in doing so, with the *shen*, which stands for mind and spirit and involves understanding the order of the cosmos[1]. Furthermore, the human tongue represents an important diagnostic medium and is a valuable instrument of examination for the well-trained physician. It is an amazing fact but nevertheless true: Not two fully identical human tongues exist on the

---

1 * Translated into Western terms, the ideograph *shen* means "giving account of the order of the cosmos."

planet. A skilful diagnosis of the tongue structures incorporates an essential supplement of a medical diagnosis, Western or Chinese, as far as the integration of the whole individual patient and her or his disease is concerned.

It must be mentioned, though, that Chinese medicine not only makes use of observing the tongue but also of viewing the patient as a whole (*wang*), of hearing and smelling (*wén*), taking the patient's history (*wèn*), and palpation (*qie*), including pulse diagnosis. A Chinese doctor's goal is to work out an individual analysis of his or her patient by differentiating the symptoms in order to find out the relevant syndrome (*bian zheng*) which is the root of each proper therapy by needle treatment, moxibustion, herbal prescriptions, and dietetics. In every single case, an additional orthodox Western diagnosis is required in order to obtain a reliable representation of clinical findings. On the other hand, practising Chinese medicine and acupuncture based only on reductionist Western diagnoses by using conventional terms such as headache, migraine, hepatitis, low pack pain, fibromyalgia, neurosis, mental depression, etc. as clinical starting points would likewise be a mere window-dressing approach. Chinese tongue diagnosis shows how erroneous it is to rely on this frequently applied Western custom alone.

Foundations

Revising and Memorizing Anatomy and Physiology

▶ Chapter 2

2 History and Scientific Foundations of Tongue Diagnosis

Historical Aspects

The inspection and evaluation of the tongue for diagnostic purposes is called **tongue diagnosis** (*she zhen*) in Chinese medicine. Tongue diagnosis is an essential part of diagnosis by observation (*wang*). This special diagnostic procedure has a long history and is based on experience gathered by Chinese physicians back in ancient times and further during the centuries and millennia. Suggestions for tongue diagnosis are given in the ***Huang-Di Nei-Ching Su-Wen*** (Chapters 32 and 37) and, especially, in the ***Ling-Shu Jing*** (Chapters 10, 23, and 37), as well as in Zhang Zhong-Jing's famous book ***Jin-Gui Yao-Lüe*** (Chapters 10 and 16), where a yellow coating is described as significant for constipation and a bluish tongue as a sign of blood stagnation.

Additional clinical experiences have been gathered in China since these early days, creating a body of continuous research which finally leads to the system of tongue diagnosis presented in the following. Chinese medical diagnosis relies on the evidence that the human tongue reflects the **totality** of healthy, as well as sick organisms, and consequently discloses the underlying causes **(ground)** of their disturbances. This can be appreciated by studying the development of the tongue in the human embryo (cf. p. 25). Thus, in order to practically apply the complete medical knowledge involved one has to first study and understand the developmental anatomy (ontogenesis) of the tongue and the physiological relationship between organism and tongue.

Relationship between Tongue, Vessel Pathways (*Jing Mai*), and Internal Organs (*Zang Fu*)

A correct rendering of the book title **Huang-Di Nei-Ching** is: "The Yellow Emperor's Treatise on the Network of Pulsating Blood Vessels under the Body's Surface in the Interior of the Organism which is Accessible by Pulse Diagnosis." Accordingly, the *jing mai* are the blood vessels, arteries, and veins, in connection with nervous pathways, all well-known structures of modern orthodox medicine. According to the original sources, the effects of needle and moxibustion therapy, as well as those of medicinal herbs are brought about via the blood vessels, lymphatic vessels, and the nervous system. Chinese pulse diagnosis was originally used to evaluate the strength or weakness of blood flow within the body's pulsating arteries, and only understood in this way does it make sense. Pulse diagnosis is referred to in many chapters of the *Huang-Di Nei-Ching*. It enables the physician to analyze the blood distribution within the circulatory system, especially before and after a patient is treated by acupuncture, moxibustion, and herbal prescriptions.

Historically, tongue diagnosis was developed later than pulse diagnosis. Chapter 32 of the *Huang-Di Nei-Jing Su-Wen* ("Needle Treatment of Heat Diseases") deals with a yellow coating of the tongue in cases revealing a hot body (fever) of a patient with lung heat disease (e. g., pneumonia). But tongue diagnosis is already frequently mentioned in the second part of the *Nei-Ching*, the *Ling-Shu Jing*, for example in Chapter 37, entitled "Five Examinations and Five Applications of the Sensory Organs and Colors," where the relationship between the tongue and the **heart** is presented:

> The condition of the heart can be analyzed and understood by an examination of the tongue.

The treasury organs lung, liver, spleen, and kidney can be evaluated in a similar way.

In this context, "heart" not only refers to the heart organ (*xin*) but also to its mental equivalent, the *shen* that includes language and speech. Chapter 10 (entitled *Jing Mai*, "The Pulsating Blood Vessels") of the same book relates the tongue to the course of the **kidney** vessel (*zu shao yin*) passing through **liver** and **lung** on its way and ending up on the root of the tongue, from where it turns back to the **heart** and **pericardium** (*luo*, vessels of the heart). Diseases of the kidney often are associated with a hot and burning mouth and a dry tongue. Accordingly, the condition of the kidney organ can be evaluated by inspecting the root of the tongue.

The **spleen** vessel (*zu tai yin*) terminates underneath the body of the tongue (inserting into the superior and inferior longitudinal, and into the transverse and vertical muscles) and branches into the inferior side of the tongue where the openings of the submandibular and sublingual glands and the lingual glands, including the anterior lingual gland, are located.

The *Ling-Shu Jing* continues:

> Lips and tongue are the foundation of the muscles; they have to receive the nutritional agents (*ying*) in order to restore the organism via the blood vessels. Whenever they become unable to do so, the vessels cannot transport the nourishing food material toward the muscles. In such a case, the blood supply of the spleen vessel (*zu tai yin*) is poor, the blood vessels get weak, the muscles become atrophic, the skin shrivels, and the whole body shrinks. The tongue of such a person gets weak and dry.

In cases of an *exterior* pathogenic influence on the spleen the root of the tongue turns rigid; in cases of an *interior* disease of the spleen organ the whole tongue becomes sore and painful.

The course of the **liver** blood vessel (*zu jue yin*) is described in the *Ling-Shu Jing* with a special branch leading upward to the cheeks and to the lips being connected with the lateral border of the tongue (in close contact with teeth and cheeks).

According to the *Ling-Shu Jing*, the tongue is in close connection with the five (or six) internal organs via the blood vessels of **heart**, **spleen**, **kidney**, and **liver**, and via additional vessels branching off toward the **lung** and the **pericardium**. Chapter 17 of the Ling-Shu Jing explains the connection between the upper burner (upper heater) and the lungs, the stomach, and the large intestine. Moreover, Chapter 10 emphasizes the connections between the whole blood vessel system and the internal organs, thus introducing an early understanding of the blood circulation. Primitive organ pathology is set out as well and this became the forerunner of the differentiating syndrome diagnosis (*bian zheng*), which to this day constitutes the basis for the clinical application of acupuncture, moxibustion, and herbal prescriptions.

According to the *Ling-Shu Jing*, the appearance of the tongue reveals a characteristic relationship with the internal organs as follows:
- The heart (*xin and shen*) corresponds to the whole tongue.
- The kidney vessels end at the root of the tongue.
- The spleen vessels enter into the body and the inferior side of the tongue.
- The liver vessels are related to the margin of the tongue.
- The lung (and the heart) vessels are connected with the tip of the tongue.
- The upper burner (or heater), the lung, large intestine, and stomach vessels are in relation with the tongue.
- The lung and the pericardium vessels are connected with the tongue via branches of the kidney vessels.

Unfortunately, the application of tongue diagnosis has been almost forgotten in modern Western medicine. We would, therefore, like to dedicate this atlas in particular to our Western medical colleagues, the conventional orthodox physicians of all specialties.

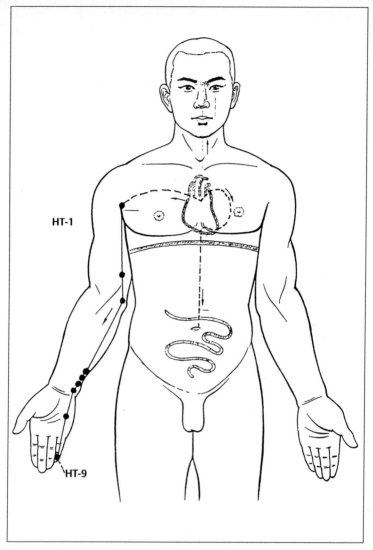

Fig. **1: The heart channel (or vessel)**

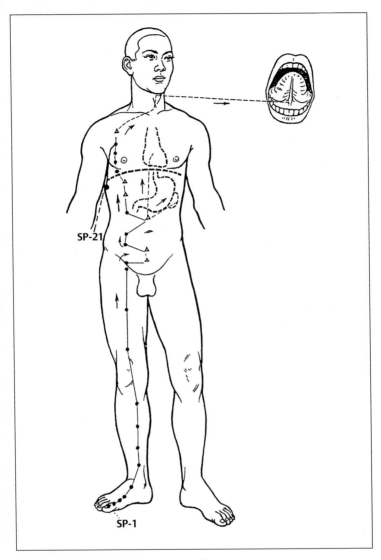

Fig. 2: The spleen channel (or vessel)

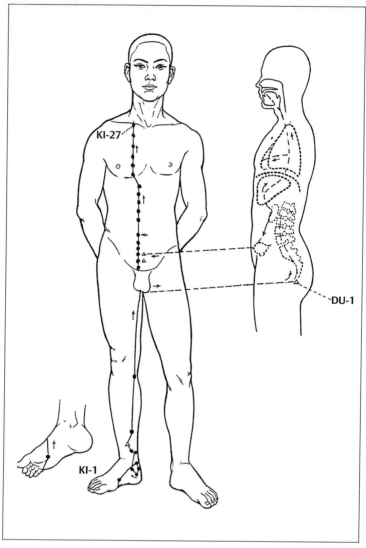

Fig. 3: **The kidney channel (or vessel)**

Basics

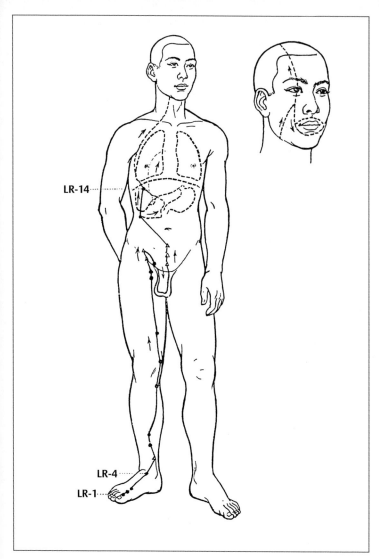

Fig. **4: The liver channel (or vessel)**

Anatomical and Physiological Foundations (Cf. Figs. 5–16)

Modern scientific tongue diagnosis is based on anatomy, embryology, histology, and pathophysiology, as well as on an understanding of the basic theories of Chinese medicine. A practitioner without such fundamental medical knowledge is unable to practise Chinese tongue diagnosis because he or she has to make do without the necessary scientific fundamentals. The substantiation of Chinese medicine by methods of orthodox Western medicine, which is nowadays required worldwide, is impressively demonstrated in the clinical evaluation of tongue diagnosis. In other words, the different diagnostic methods of both medicines, Western and Chinese, must be amalgamated to create the New Medical Paradigm, the starting point of a new Global Medicine based on an encompassing medical logic.

The Structure of the Tongue

The tongue consists of the body, the root, the back, the lower side connected with the floor of the mouth, the margin, and the tip. The back of the tongue is covered with the **lingual mucosa**, which is formed by six types of different lingual papillae (papillae linguales) described below.

The Lingual Papillae

The following types of mucosal structures (papillae) can be distinguished:

1. Filiform papillae	→ Very slender, almost threadlike epithelial elevations on connective tissue sockets. They are often split at their end and located on the tip and in the middle of the tongue.
2. Conical papillae	→ A special type of filiform papillae, somewhat larger and longer, with conical ends bent backward.
3. Fungiform papillae	→ Mushroomlike and flattened on top.
4. Circumvallated papillae	→ Seven to twelve rather large papillae, round in cross section, located in front of the terminal sulcus. Taste buds lie in the circular groove surrounding them.
5. Lentiform papillae	→ Short fungiform papillae.
6. Foliate papillae	→ Several parallel mucosal folds bearing taste buds located along the posterolateral border of the tongue.

The Muscles of the Tongue

Morphology of the Tongue Muscles

The body of the tongue consists of eight muscles: Four skeleton muscles (*musculi skleleti*) and four proper, cruciate, or cutaneous muscles. The motoric innervation of all eight muscles is by the hypoglossal nerve (cranial nerve XII).

The four skeleton muscles (*musculi skleleti*) of the tongue

1. Genioglossus muscle ➔ Originates at the mental spine of the mandible and inserts fan-shaped on the lower side of the tongue from tip to base.
▷ Action: Draws the tongue forward toward the chin. Its anterior fibers bend the tip of the tongue downward.

2. Hyoglossus muscle ➔ Originates at the body and the greater horn of the hyoid bone and radiates into the lateral portions of the tongue as far as the mucous membrane.
▷ Action: Draws the base of the tongue down and backward.

3. Chondroglossus muscle ➔ Originates at the lesser horn of the hyoid bone and radiates into the lateral portion of the tongue as far as the mucous membrane.
▷ Action: Draws the tongue backward and downward.

4. Styloglossus muscle ➔ Originates from the styloid process and radiates from behind and above into the lateral portions

of the tongue and interlaces with the fibers of the hyoglossus muscle.
▷ Action: Draws the tongue backward and upward.

The four cruciate or cutaneous muscles

5. Superior longitudinal muscle → Muscle bundles directly beneath the mucous membrane, extending from the tip of the tongue into the area of the hyoid bone.
▷ Action: Shortens the tongue.

6. Inferior longitudinal muscle → System of fibers very close to the inferior side of the tongue extending from base to tip.
▷ Action: Shortens the tongue and modulates its shape.

7. Transverse muscle of the tongue → Muscle fibers between the longitudinal fiber system. They originate from the septum of the tongue and insert into the mucous membranes on the sides of the tongue.
▷ Action: Extends the tongue together with the vertical fibers of the vertical muscle. In addition, it constricts and rounds the tongue.

8. Vertical muscle of the tongue → Muscle fibers running from the dorsum of the tongue to the inferior surface.
▷ Action: Flattens the tongue.

Physiological Effect of the Tongue Muscles

The great plasticity of the tongue is brought about by the three-dimensional structure of its muscles. Especially the interior muscles enable the tongue to assume a quite varied shape. The longitudinal muscles shorten the tongue, the vertical muscles flatten it, and the transverse fibers narrow and round it. The skeleton muscles (*musculi skeleti*) mainly change the position of the tongue; in addition, they contribute to a changing of its shape. The styloglossus and the hyoglossus muscles draw the tongue backward. The first brings it upward, the second downward. The posterior fibers of the genioglossus draw the base of the tongue forward; its central fibers draw the body of the tongue forward and downward, away from the palate. The anterior fibers of the genioglossus bend the tip of the tongue downward. Thus, by changing the shape and position of the tongue the tip can reach any point in the oral cavity. Furthermore, the tongue can be stretched and stuck far out of the mouth widely by an interplay of the genioglossus, the transverse, and the vertical muscles. In sticking out the tongue, the genioglossus draws the tongue forward; the transverse and vertical muscles lengthen the tongue.

The tongue conveys food toward the molar teeth for chewing and supports the formation of food bolus, including salivation and lubrication. The large internal surface of the gastrointestinal tract (roughly $100 \, m^2$) requires a very effective immune defense system. Saliva contains *mucins*, *immunoglobulin A*, and *lysozyme* that prevent the penetration of pathogens. The solid food is chewed and mixed with saliva. The esophagus rapidly transports the food bolus to the stomach. The mucosa of the tongue serves as a sensory organ for tasting (cf. p. 14). Furthermore, the tongue has an important function in the production of sound and for the articulation of human language.

Additional Structures of the Tongue

1. Septum of the tongue
2. Lingual aponeurosis
3. Median sulcus
4. Deep lingual artery
5. Sublingual artery
6. Deep lingual vein
7. Sublingual vein
8. Terminal sulcus
9. Foramen cecum linguae
10. Lingual follicles (folliculi linguales). These are rounded mucosal elevations, 1–5 mm in diameter, caused by underlying lymphatic tissue. Each has a crypt in its center. Altogether they form the lingual tonsil.

Arterial Supply of the Tongue (Cf. fig. 8 and 9)

The tongue is supplied with oxygenated ("arterialized") blood via the external carotid artery. On the level of the greater horn of the hyoid bone the lingual artery branches off from it as its second anterior branch. It extends sinuously to the tip of the tongue, covered laterally by the hyoglossus muscle. The deep lingual artery is the main branch of the lingual artery running between genioglossus and inferior longitudinal muscles to the tip of the tongue. It anastomoses with the fellow artery of the opposite side.

Veins of the Tongue

The venous drainage of the tongue is via the lingual vein located near the lingual artery. It empties into the internal jugular vein. Patients with a resistance in their pulmonary circulation show a damming-up of venous blood, resulting in visible and enlarged veins on the margin and the inferior side of the tongue. In such a case the two deep lingual veins underneath the tongue become thickened and dark blue or purple in color.

Lymphatic Vessels of the Tongue (Cf. fig. 11c)

The following lymphatic vessels and lymph nodes are connected with the tongue:

1. Submandibular lymph nodes	→ Located between the mandible and the submandibular gland.
2. Buccinator lymph node	→ Located deep on the buccinator muscle.
3. Submental lymph nodes	→ Two or three small nodes located between the frontal bellies of the digastric muscles.
4. Jugulodigastric node	→ Located between omohyoid muscle and internal jugular vein.
5. Deep cervical lymph nodes	→ A group of nodes located at the side of the throat. They represent the second filter station for almost all head and neck lymph nodes

The Nerves of the Tongue

1. The mandibular nerve. It is the third division of the trigeminal nerve (cranial nerve V), passing through the oval foramen into the infratemporal fossa. It contains sensory and motor fibers for the masticatory muscles.
2. Intermediate nerve (Wrisberg nerve). Nonmotor part of the facial nerve (VII). It arises separately from the brain stem between facial and vestibulocochlear nerves and carries autonomic and taste fibers. Joins the facial nerve after various anastomoses inside the petrosal bone.
3. Chorda tympani (from VII). It consists of parasympathetic fibers for the submandibular ganglion and sensory fibers from taste

buds of the anterior two thirds of the tongue. The chorda tympani connects the intermediate nerve (from VII) with the lingual nerve (from V3).

4. Glossopharyngeal nerve (IX). It contains lingual branches with sensory (taste) fibers for the mucosa of the posterior third of the tongue, including the circumvallate papillae. The lingual nerve (from V3) supplies it in addition via the chorda tympani (from VII).

5. The pharyngeal branches of the vagus nerve (X) radiate into the pharyngeal plexus, a nerve network under the middle constrictor of the pharynx composed of the glossopharyngeal and vagus nerves and the cervical sympathetic trunk. A thin branch of the pharyngeal plexus supplies the tongue and the autonomic fibers of the external carotid plexus.

6. The motor nerve of the tongue is the hypoglossal nerve (XII). It passes through the hypoglossal canal and continues anteriorly between internal jugular vein and anterior carotid artery to the posterior margin of the floor of the mouth and to the tongue. Its lingual branches innervate the hyoglossus, styloglossus, genioglossus, chondroglossus, and the intrinsic muscles of the tongue.

Gustatory Pathways, Sense of Taste, and Pain Perception

Sensory stimuli from the taste buds are conducted to endings of the **glossopharyngeal** (IX), **facial** (VII, intermediate nerve and chorda tympani), and **vagus** (X) cranial nerves. The glossopharyngeal nerve supplies the circumvallated and the foliate papillae. The intermediate nerve in connection with the chorda tympani and the lingual nerve (from V3) conduct the taste sensation from the fungiform papillae. The vagus nerve supplies taste buds located on the posterior part of the dorsum of the tongue (radix linguae) and at the entrance of the pharynx.

Taste buds consist of clusters of 50–100 secondary sensory cells on the tongue, which are renewed in a two-week cycle. Humans have around 5000 taste buds. Children and younger humans have multiple taste buds, they diminish gradually during life, so that older people possess fewer taste buds. Taste buds can disappear during certain diseases, but can grow again if the necessary stimuli for regrowth are transmitted to the tongue by the cranial nerves involved.

Taste stimuli are relayed by the *nucleus tractus solitarii* and converge on the postcentral (sensory) gyrus of the cortex via the thalamus, the hypothalamus, and the pons.

Qualities of taste are defined as sweet, sour, salty, and bitter. The specific taste sensor cells for these qualities are distributed over the whole tongue but differ with respect to their density. *Umami*, the taste sensation caused by monosodium L-glutamate (MSG), is now classified as a fifth quality of taste. *Umami* is mainly found in protein-rich food. Sweet food is mainly tasted with the tip, salty with the tip and the margin, sour with the margin, and bitter (glossopharyngeal nerve) with the posterior part, the root of the tongue (radix linguae) (cf. Fig. 16).

The sense of taste has a protective function, as spoiled or bitter-tasting food (related to a low taste threshold) is often poisonous. Tasting substances also stimulates the secretion of saliva and of gastric juices. Among other components, saliva contains *immunoglobulin* A and *lysozyme*, which are part of the immune defense system, referred to as *wei* in Chinese medicine.

Sensations of pain, heat, and touch are conducted centrally from the anterior two thirds of the tongue via the lingual nerve (from the mandibular nerve, the inferior branch of the trigeminal nerve V), and they are transmitted from the posterior third by the glossopharyngeal and the vagus nerves.

Salivary Glands and Saliva

1. The sublingual gland is a primarily mucous gland with the greater and smaller sublingual ducts. The greater opens beside the submandibular duct on the sublingual caruncula on the inferior side of the tongue. The smaller consists of approximately 40 small ducts of the sublingual gland opening on the sublingual fold and the sublingual caruncula.
2. Anterior lingual gland (Nuhn gland). A mixed gland in the tip of the tongue, with several ducts on the inferior surface.
3. The submandibular gland, a predominantly serous gland with the submandibular (or Wharton) duct, which is accompanied by glandular substance and winds around the posterior border of the mylohyoid muscle. It opens on the sublingual caruncula.
4. Lingual glands. These are a large number of mucous, serous, and mixed glands on the lateral and posterior surfaces of the tongue.
5. Although the parotid gland is not directly related to structures of the tongue it plays an important part in the secretion of saliva. It is located behind and on the ramus of the mandible. The parotid (or Stensen) duct extends from the anterior border of the masseter muscle and opens opposite the second upper molar.

Secretion of saliva

The rate of secretion of saliva from the salivary glands varies from 0.1–4 mL per minute, depending on the degree of stimulation. This adds up to about 0.5–1.5 L per day. Ninety-five percent of this is secreted by the parotid (serous saliva) and submandibular gland (mucin-rich saliva). The rest comes from the sublingual gland and from glands in the buccal mucosa.

Its constituents reflect the functions of saliva. *Mucins* serve to lubricate the food, making it easier to swallow, and to keep the mouth moist to facilitate masticator and speech-related movement. Saliva dissolves compounds in food, which is a prerequisite for taste bud stimulation and for dental and oral hygiene. Saliva has a low NaCl concentration and is hypotonic, making it suitable for rinsing of taste receptors while eating. Saliva also contains α-amylase, which starts the digestion of starches in the mouth, while *immunoglobulin* A and *lysozyme* are part of the immune defense system. The saliva secretion is very dependent on the body water content. A low content results in decreased saliva secretion. Then the tongue, mouth, and throat become dry, thereby evoking the sensation of thirst. This is an important mechanism for maintaining the fluid balance in the organism.

The Floor of the Mouth and the Inferior Side of the Tongue

When the tip of the tongue is turned upward the cavity of the mouth and the floor of the mouth become visible. The mucous membrane on the inferior surface is smooth and of a purplish color. In the medium plane it is connected to the floor of the mouth by the frenulum linguae. On each side of the frenulum small elevations of mucous membrane show up: the openings of the submandibular and sublingual ducts. Lateral to the frenulum, the deep lingual vein is visible through the mucous membrane, and at the lateral side of the vein there is a fringed fold of mucous membrane, the fimbriated fold (*plica fimbriata*), which is directed forward and medially toward the tip of the tongue. Underneath this fold is the sublingual gland. In humans with a damming-back of the pulmonary circulation the deep lingual veins become dark blue or purple in color, then the dorsum of the tongue may assume a purple color, too. For Chinese diagnostics this reveals a blockage of blood (*yu xue*). A bluish color of the tongue can also reveal a general lack of oxygen.

Tongue Development in the Embryo (Fig. 16)

The development of the tongue involves all components of the pharyngeal (or branchial) arches and takes place at the same time as the development of the pharyngeal (branchial) arch nerves, the aortic arches, and the visceral skeleton in the embryo. The developing tongue bulges at the floor of the pharynx behind the pharyngeal membrane and grows interiorly into the oral cavity (Fig. **16a**). It consists of parts of the first, second, and third pharyngeal arches. The site of the origin of the thyroid gland is the remaining foramen cecum at the base of the tongue. It marks the original boundary between the first and second arches (Fig. **16b**). In fish, the pharyngeal arches develop into branchial arches. That is why the pharyngeal arches were named branchial arches in the older anatomical literature.

The lingual mucosa develops from the first to fourth pharyngeal arches on the floor of the oral cavity. The first to appear is the single median tongue bud (middle lingual swelling), posterior to which the tuberculum impar (or tuberculum hyoideum) develops, whose endodermal epithelium gives rise to the primordial thyroid tissue. The remaining foramen cecum marks the location of the former thyreoglossal duct after its closure.

A little later, two oval distal tongue buds (or lingual swellings) appear on the endodermal aspect of the mandibular processes. They meet each other in front, converge on the median tongue bud, and constitute the **anterior** or **oral part** of the tongue, which is later separated from the pharyngeal part by the terminal sulcus. Posterior to the tuberculum impar the second, third, and fourth pharyngeal arches form a median tongue bud, the hypobranchial eminence (or copula of His), which results in the pharyngeal floor and the root (pharyngeal part) of the tongue.

The relation of the tongue to the pharyngeal arches remains apparent in the arrangement of the **tongue musculature** (cf. p. 16f.): The genioglossus muscle originates at the genu of the mandible, which is derived from the first pharyngeal arch. The styloglossus muscle arises from the styloid process, a part of the second pharyngeal arch. The hyoglossus originates from the hyoid bone, which arises from the second and third arches. The tongue musculature is derived from myoblasts of the occipital myotome that migrate into the tongue in broad tracts. They receive their motor innervation from the hypoglossal nerve (XII).

The relations to the three pharyngeal arches are also apparent in the composite **sensory nerve supply** of the tongue. Sensory impulses from the anterior oral part are mediated by

(a) The lingual nerve of the first branchial arch (mandibular nerve V3), and
(b) By the chorda tympani (from facial nerve VII) derived from the second branchial arch.
(c) The **posterior**, pharyngeal **part** of the tongue is innervated by the glossopharyngeal, the nerve of the third branchial arch.

The fourth pharyngeal arch supplies the vagus nerve, which extends the internal branch of its superior laryngeal nerve to the postsulcal part (portion dorsal to the terminal sulcus) of the tongue.

Functional Correlation of Tongue Structures

The modifications, changes, and interrelationships of the body, the coating, and the consistency of the tongue are thus based on the development of the tongue in the human embryo. After birth, physiological and pathological changes reflecting the combined internal and external influxes are detectable on the following anatomical structures:

- The lingual mucosa and the papillae,
- The muscles of the tongue,
- The nerves of the tongue,
- The arteries and veins of the tongue,
- The lymph vessels of the tongue,
- The salivary glands of the tongue, including the secretion of saliva.

Illustrated Anatomical Structures (Figs. 6–16)

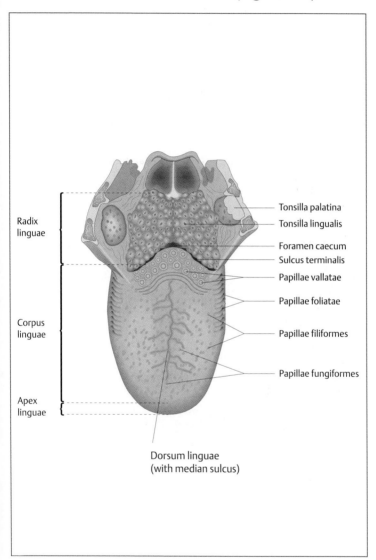

Radix linguae

Corpus linguae

Apex linguae

Tonsilla palatina
Tonsilla lingualis
Foramen caecum
Sulcus terminalis
Papillae vallatae
Papillae foliatae
Papillae filiformes
Papillae fungiformes

Dorsum linguae
(with median sulcus)

Fig. **5**: **Anatomical structures of the body of the tongue** (dorsum and root)

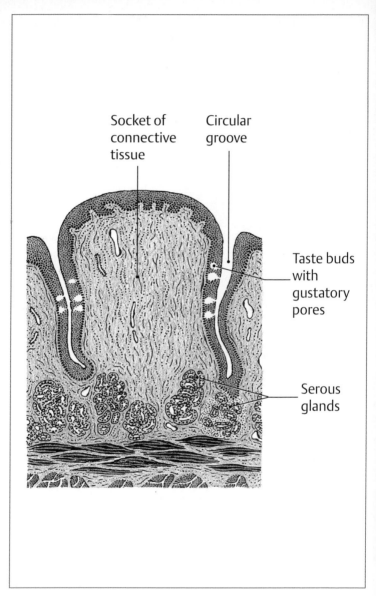

Socket of connective tissue

Circular groove

Taste buds with gustatory pores

Serous glands

Fig. **6**: **Papilla vallata** (schematic drawing)

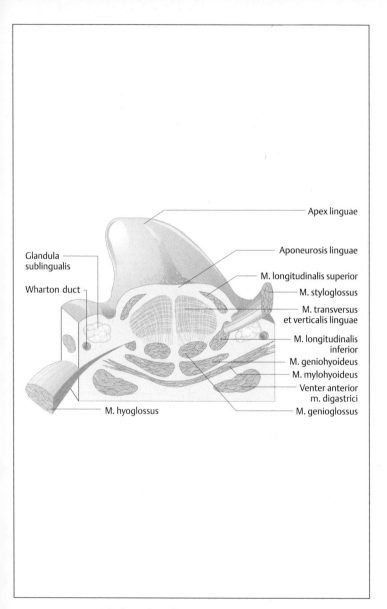

Apex linguae

Aponeurosis linguae

M. longitudinalis superior

M. styloglossus

M. transversus
et verticalis linguae

M. longitudinalis
inferior

M. geniohyoideus

M. mylohyoideus

Venter anterior
m. digastrici

M. genioglossus

Glandula
sublingualis

Wharton duct

M. hyoglossus

Fig. 7: **Extrinsic (skeleton) and intrinsic (cutaneous) muscles of the tongue**

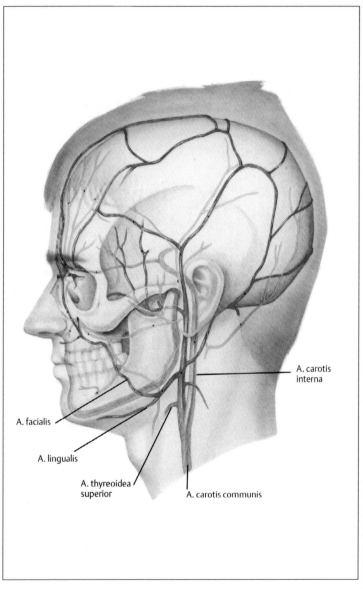

A. carotis
interna

A. facialis

A. lingualis

A. thyreoidea
superior

A. carotis communis

Fig. **8**: **Arteries of the head**

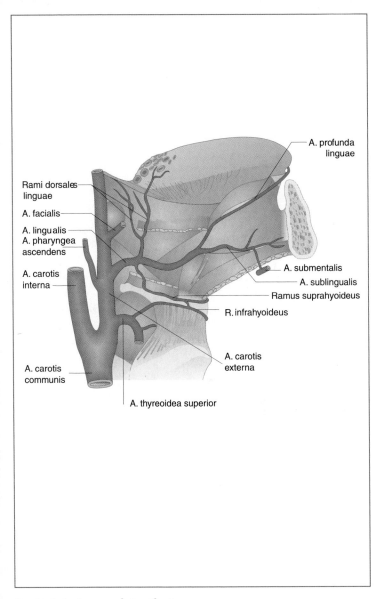

A. profunda linguae

Rami dorsales linguae

A. facialis

A. lingualis

A. pharyngea ascendens

A. carotis interna

A. carotis communis

A. submentalis

A. sublingualis

Ramus suprahyoideus

R. infrahyoideus

A. carotis externa

A. thyreoidea superior

Fig. **9**: **Arteries supplying the tongue**

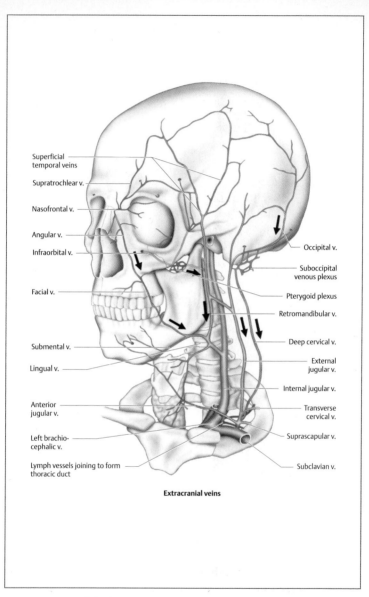

Superficial
temporal veins

Supratrochlear v.

Nasofrontal v.

Angular v.

Infraorbital v.

Facial v.

Submental v.

Lingual v.

Anterior
jugular v.

Left brachio-
cephalic v.

Lymph vessels joining to form
thoracic duct

Occipital v.

Suboccipital
venous plexus

Pterygoid plexus

Retromandibular v.

Deep cervical v.

External
jugular v.

Internal jugular v.

Transverse
cervical v.

Suprascapular v.

Subclavian v.

Extracranial veins

Fig. **10**: **Veins of the head**

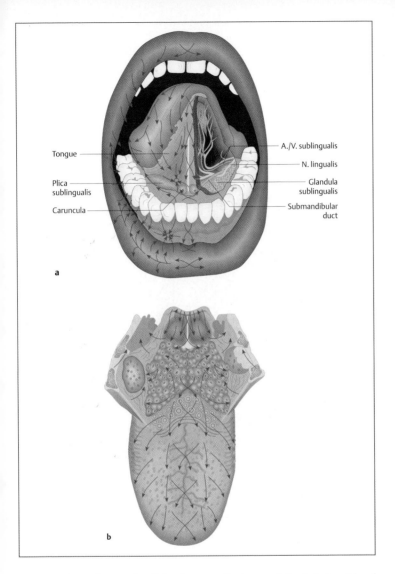

Tongue

Plica
sublingualis

Caruncula

A./V. sublingualis

N. lingualis

Glandula
sublingualis

Submandibular
duct

a

b

Fig. **11a**: **Lymph vessels of the tongue.** Drainage of the inferior side of
the tongue, of the floor of the mouth, the gums, and lips

Fig. **11b**: **Lymph vessels of the tongue.** Drainage of the dorsum and the
root of the tongue (main direction of lymphatic flow marked by arrows;
after Werner 1993, 1995)

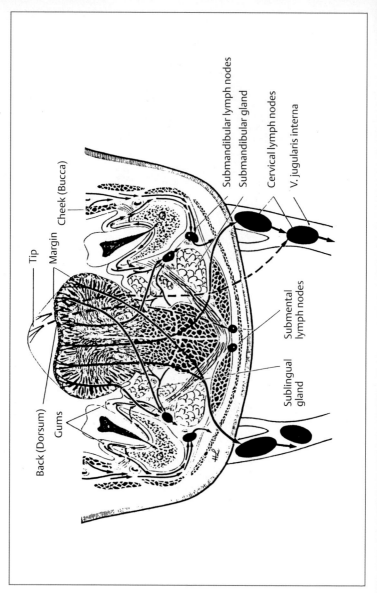

Fig. **11c**: **Lymphatic ducts and regional lymphatic nodes of the tongue** (Direction of flow marked by arrows)

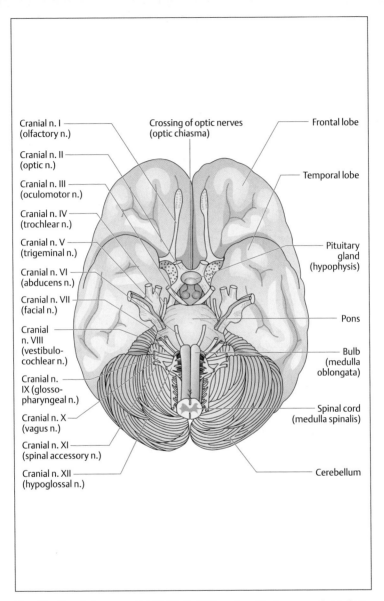

Fig. **12: Cranial nerves V, VII, IX, X, XII involved in tongue physiology**

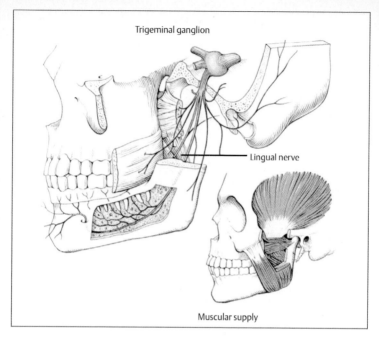

Fig. **13a:** **Important nerves of the tongue: mandibular nerve (V3)**

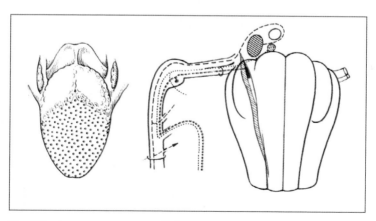

Fig. **13b:** **Important nerves of the tongue: intermediate nerve (VII) (Wrisberg nerve)**

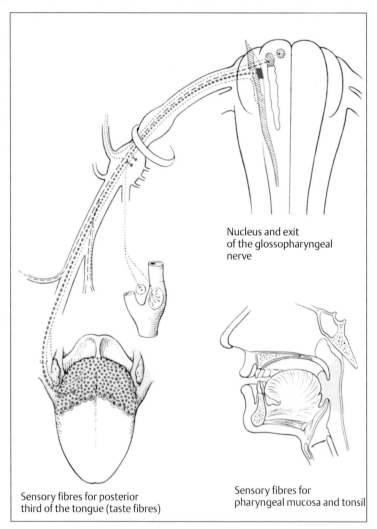

Nucleus and exit
of the glossopharyngeal
nerve

Sensory fibres for posterior
third of the tongue (taste fibres)

Sensory fibres for
pharyngeal mucosa and tonsil

Fig. **13c**: **Important nerves of the tongue: glossopharyngeal nerve (IX)**

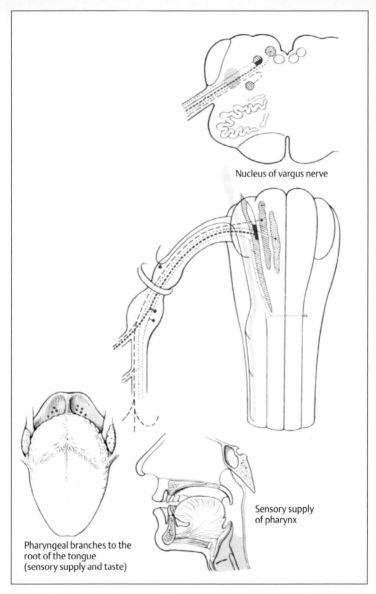

Nucleus of vargus nerve

Sensory supply
of pharynx

Pharyngeal branches to the
root of the tongue
(sensory supply and taste)

Fig. **13d: Important nerves of the tongue: vagus nerve (X)**

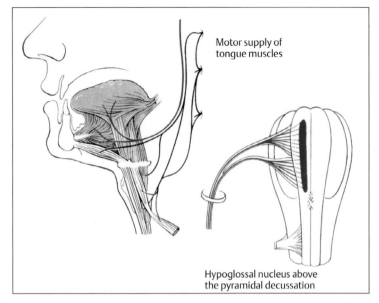

Motor supply of
tongue muscles

Hypoglossal nucleus above
the pyramidal decussation

Fig. **13e**: **Important nerves of the tongue: the hypoglossal nerve (XII)**

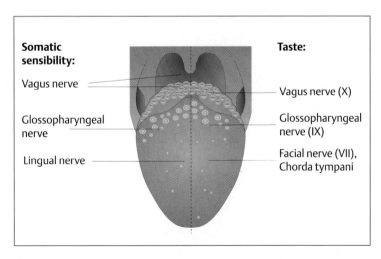

Somatic sensibility:

Vagus nerve

Glossopharyngeal nerve

Lingual nerve

Taste:

Vagus nerve (X)

Glossopharyngeal nerve (IX)

Facial nerve (VII), Chorda tympani

Fig. **14**: **Gustatory innervation and somatic sensibility**

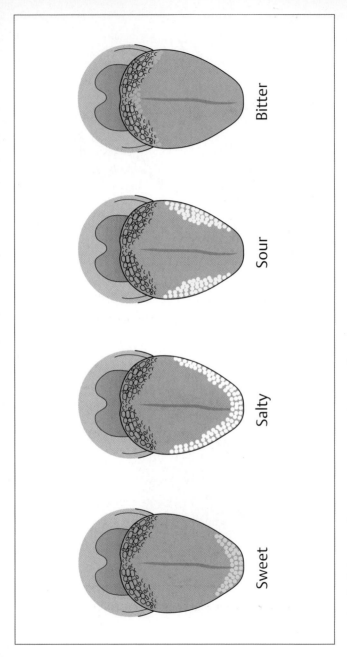

Fig. 15: **The location of various taste sensations on the tongue**

Sweet   Salty   Sour   Bitter

    Basics

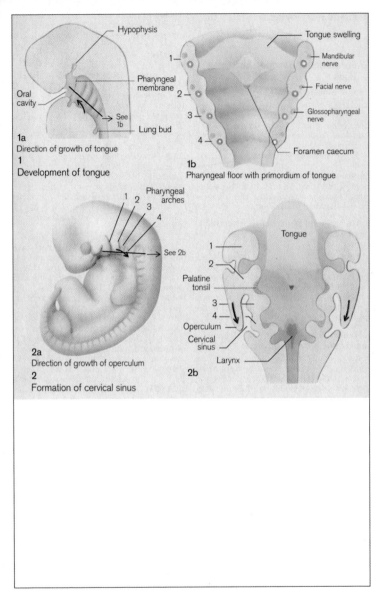

Fig. **16**: **Tongue development in the embryo.** Tongue and cervical sinus

Methodology of Tongue Diagnosis

Systematic Procedure Involving the Body, the Coating, and the Consistency of the Tongue

▶ Chapters 3 and 4

3 The Technique of Tongue Diagnosis

The patient's face is turned to the light and the tongue is examined in a flat, stretched out position, not, however, to the extent that its natural color changes. It is best to examine the tongue by daylight. If, under certain conditions, the examination has to be done by artificial light, the wrong results may be obtained. If the tongue has to be examined initially by artificial light, it is advisable to examine it again later on by daylight. It is important to distinguish between the true color of the tongue and a discoloration caused by certain foods, medication, or mechanical influences. Milk, for instance, leaves a white coating on the surface of the tongue, coffee a brown surface. Bilberries (blueberries) and beet tinge the tongue bluish-red, whereas colored sweets make the tongue look green, yellow, or blue. Chocolate leaves a brown smear; toothpaste can leave a white layer, etc. The coating on the tongue can also be changed by brushing it with a toothbrush or after eating certain kinds of food. Food can be responsible for rubbing off a thick coating and thus make the coating look thinner or even normal. Hot, pungent, and spicy food can change the color of the tongue, leaving it either bright red or dark purple. For these reasons, the physician should never examine the tongue immediately after the patient has eaten, drunk, or brushed his or her teeth and tongue.

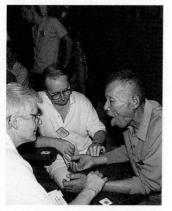

Fig. **17**

4 Systematic Procedure of Tongue Diagnosis

The basic method of any medical examination is the differentiation between opposed phenomena. In Chinese medicine this procedure is called *bian zheng*, which is the differentiation between contradictory findings. It is the Chinese version of the famous Principle of Contradiction, which for occidental science was formulated by the Greek philosophers Heraclitus, Parmenides, Plato, and Aristotle.

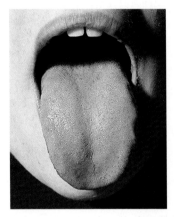

Fig. **18**

In examining the tongue the physician must be able to differentiate between the body of the tongue and the coating. In addition, the structure or consistency of the tongue is important. The body of the tongue is made up of the tongue muscles, arteries and veins, lymphatic vessels, salivary glands, and fine blood vessels (capillaries). The coating is the uppermost layer of the tongue. Usually, the human tongue looks soft and tender and moves freely and easily. It is light red, slightly wet, and covered with a fine white layer. Chinese medicine refers to this normal appearance of the tongue as a "light red tongue with a thin white coating (Fig. **18**)."

This normal condition of the tongue changes with the seasons and climate. In summer the coating is usually somewhat thicker or it turns yellow as the result of summer heat. In autumn the coating is thin, white, and slightly dry. The physician must be aware of these natural seasonal changes so as not to confuse them with pathological ones.

In the case of illness, changes in the body of the tongue must be differentiated from changes in the coating of the tongue. The body of the tongue can undergo changes in consistency, color, and form. It primarily reflects either strength or weakness of the arterial or venous blood flow (*xue qi*), increased or decreased capillary pressure and lymph drainage, decreased concentration of plasma proteins, etc. In Chinese medicine this is referred to as a deficiency or a fullness of the vessels of storage and hollow organs, the *jing mai*, running deep inside the organism. The coating of the tongue can change in form, color, and in consistency as well. This will indicate whether the disease is more superficial or internal and also reflects the relationship between the patient's power of resistance (*zheng*) and the external disturbance (*xie*).

Chinese medicine divides the tongue into four areas:
- The **tip**,
- The **center**,
- The **root** or base, and
- The **sides** (margin).

Tongue areas and organ diseases:
- Diseases of the **heart** and **lungs** can be detected by the condition of the tip.
- The center of the tongue reflects the condition of the **spleen** and **stomach**.
- The root or base corresponds to the **kidneys**, the **bladder**, and **intestines**.
- The sides of the tongue refer to the **liver** and **gallbladder**.

If this method of division is applied to the levels of three burners (three heaters or "energizers"), then
- The tip of the tongue corresponds to the upper burner,
- The middle section of the tongue to the middle burner, and
- The base to the lower burner.

According to this arrangement, the Chinese physician can diagnose disorders related to the internal organs.

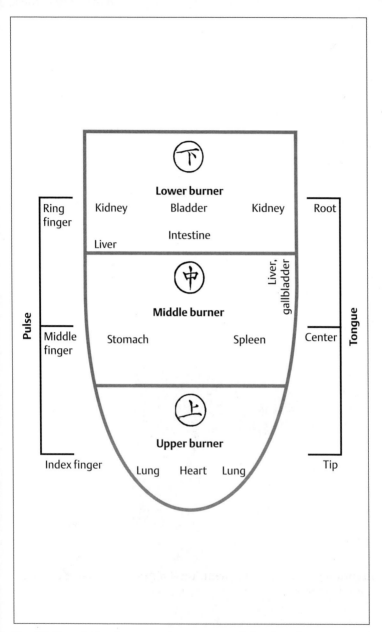

Fig. **19**: **Correlation between the tongue and the three burners**

The Body of the Tongue

Color of the Tongue Body

Criteria
- Normal
- Light, white
- Red
- Dark red
- Greenish-purple

1. Normal color of the tongue body

A normal tongue is pink, soft, flexible, slightly wet, and covered with a thin whitish layer, which cannot even be called a "coating." A patient with such a tongue is not seriously ill. One comes across such a tongue in cases of mild infectious diseases which have affected the organism only superficially (Fig. **20**).

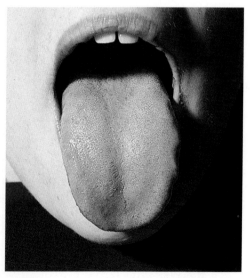

Fig. **20**

2. The light, white tongue

The color of such a tongue is definitely lighter than the normal. It corresponds to a cold and deficiency condition, which is usually a sign of weakness in the *yang* function (*yang qi*) and of an insufficiency of blood supply (Fig. **21**).

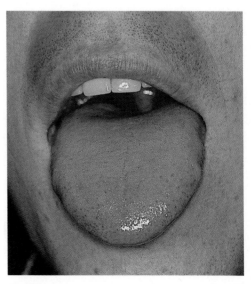

Fig. **21**

3. The red tongue

This tongue is bright red and overall noticeably darker than the normal tongue. Such a tongue corresponds to a heat condition and is usually a sign of an internal heat fullness syndrome. It can also be a sign of a *yin* deficiency associated with ascending internal fire (Fig. **22**).

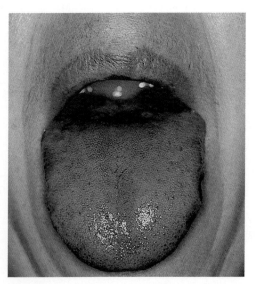

Fig. **22**

4. The dark red tongue

This corresponds to a condition of extreme heat. It usually denotes a case of infectious heat disease whereby a heat disturbance has caused the pathological conditions of *ying fen* or *xue fen* syndrome. These are serious and often life-threatening conditions (Fig. **23**).

If this type of tongue appears in a patient who is chronically ill, it indicates a *yin* deficiency with extreme fire. The deeper the color of the red or dark red tongue, the stronger is the influence of the pathological heat disturbance. In this patient, a former, long-term drug addict, the central furrow runs as far as the tip, splitting it into two halves and indicating a serious disorder of the heart (Fig. **24**).

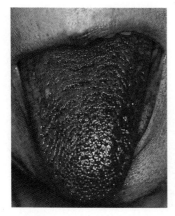
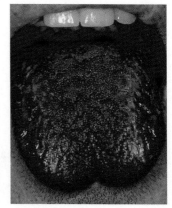

Fig. **23**   Fig. **24**

5. The blue-greenish and purple tongue

The color is greenish-purple as a whole or it displays purple or greenish patches or spots. This means that the organism is suffering from the effects of heat or cold. If the greenish-purple color is noticeably dark and the tongue is dry or just slightly moist, this is a pronounced heat effect. If the color is light and the tongue is very wet, this indicates a stagnation of blood (*yu xue*).

I treated this Chinese patient in 1977 at the *Hua-Dong* Hospital in Shanghai. She suffered from a deficiency of blood coagulation as a result of thrombocytopenia, which led to multiple bleeding into her joints (hemarthrosis) with severe joint pain. Chinese medicine refers to this condition as blood stagnation (Fig. **25**).

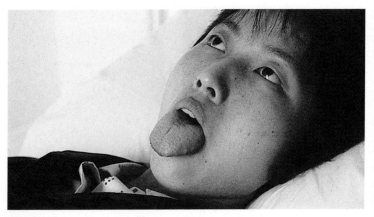

Fig. **25**

A purple tongue can either indicate an external influence of cold or an internal heat influence. In order to distinguish these two conditions, it should be noted whether the tongue is dry and its color dark (internal heat with blood stagnation) (Fig. **26**).

If the color fo the body is lighter and the tongue is wet this indicates a cold disturbance associated with a stagnation of *qi* and blood (Fig. **27**).

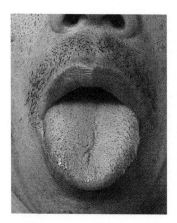

Fig. **26**

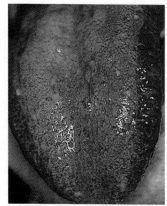

Fig. **27**

The Shape of the Body

Criteria

- ■ Wrinkled, rough
- ■ Tender, fine
- ■ Swollen
- ■ Thin, small
- ■ Fissured
- ■ Tooth marks
- ■ Granular

1. The wrinkled, rough tongue

Chinese medicine refers to the wrinkled, rough tongue with numerous grooves as an "old" (*lao*) tongue. It corresponds to a fullness syndrome or a heat syndrome, or a diminished essence (*jing*) and is frequently seen in older people. (Fig. **28**). The tongue of the woman shown in Figure **29** presents numerous reddened foliate papillae on its tip as a sign of fire in the upper burner, in this case in the heart; she suffers from mild insomnia and nervousness.

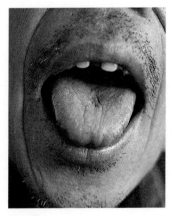

Fig. **28**

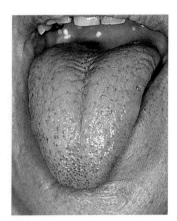

Fig. **29**

2. The tender and fine tongue

Such a tongue is referred to as a "young" (*nen*) tongue; it indicates a mild deficiency and cold condition. The tongue presented in Figure **30** is more or less still normal; it just shows a slight *yang* deficiency and an influence of cold.

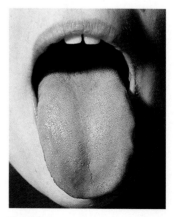

Fig. **30**

3. The swollen tongue

It is larger and thicker than the normal tongue (Fig. **31**).

If the color of the swollen tongue is light and white, this is a sign of an emptiness of *yang* in the spleen and stomach. This female patient, in addition, presents tooth marks on both sides of her tongue which are quite typical for a *yang* deficiency (Fig. **32**).

If the swollen tongue is red, it shows that there is an internal heat or a profuse disturbing heat with a deficiency of *yin* inside the organism. The tooth marks reveal a simultaneous *yang* deficiency (Fig. **33**).

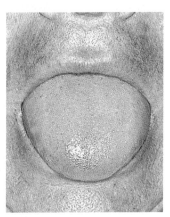

Fig. **31**

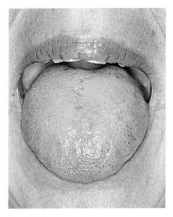

Fig. **32**

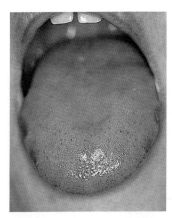

Fig. **33**

4. The thin, small tongue

A thin, small tongue which is light in color usually indicates a deficiency of blood and qi (*xue qi*) or it indicates that both heart and spleen are in a condition of emptiness. Such a condition can often be found in younger individuals with psychosomatic disorder (lack of appetite, insomnia, forgetfulness, nervousness, palpitation, etc.) (Fig. **34**).

A dark red, thin, small tongue corresponds to a *yin* emptiness with an abundance of heat, rendering the body fluids (*jin ye*) diminished or impaired. This is usually a sign of a serious disease. The patient depicted in Figure **35** is a rather tall person but his tongue is not at all in proportion with his body height of 189 cm. He suffers from high blood pressure, insomnia, and diabetes due to *yin* deficiency and internal heat.

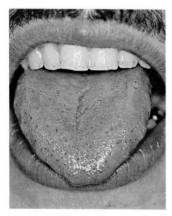

Fig. **34**

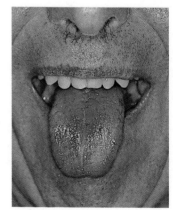

Fig. **35**

5. The fissured tongue

If the tongue has many transverse and longitudinal fissures with cracks and grooves in it, it is referred to as a "fissured tongue." If such a tongue is also dark red, this usually shows the presence of an abundance of heat. The patient in Figure **36** suffers from a severe and generalized allergy.

If such a tongue is white and light in appearance, this can indicate a lack of *yin* and blood. The patient shown in Figure **37** suffers from multiple disorders of his gastrointestinal tract and has a history of hepatitis.

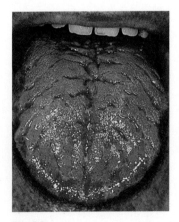

Fig. **36**

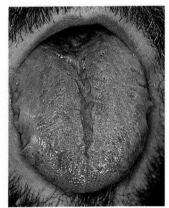

Fig. **37**

6. The tongue with tooth marks

Tooth marks on the edges of the tongue are usually found in a swollen tongue. The teeth press against the tongue because it has become too large for the oral cavity. This is presented especially by patients suffering from a deficiency of the *yang qi* with cold symptoms (Fig. **38**, **39**).

Such a tongue can develop rapidly, in cases of severe exhaustion even within a few hours. After the person recovers the tongue gets back to normal quickly.

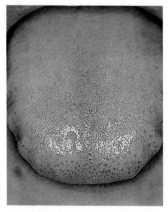

Fig. **38**

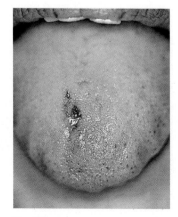

Fig. **39**

7. The granular tongue

Such a tongue appears when the filiform papillae get larger and thicker than normal or when they are converted into fungiform papillae. A granular tongue usually suggests a profuse, severe external heat disturbance inside the organism (Fig. **40**). The more intense the external heat, the larger the red grains on the tongue. If these appear on the tip of the tongue, it is a sign of abundant heart–fire (Fig. **41**).

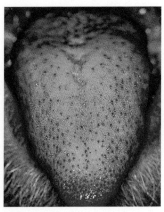

Fig. **40**

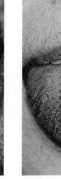

Fig. **41**

If the granules are located on the sides of the tongue, this indicates abundant fire in the liver and gallbladder (Fig. **42**). If they show up in the middle of the tongue, this is a sign of an abundant heat in the spleen, stomach, and intestines (Fig. **42**). The more the granular papillae move towards the tip of the tongue, the more severe is the implication of the upper burner (heart, lungs, pericardium), as shown in Figure **43**.

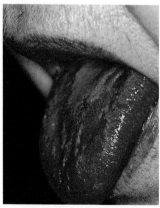

Fig. **42**

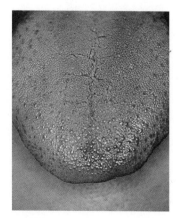

Fig. **43**

The Consistency of the Tongue

Criteria
- Weak, frail
- Hard, stiff
- Slanting
- Shortened, shrunken
- Trembling
- Protruding (stretched out) and restless

1. The weak, frail tongue

This tongue is weak and without strength. It is unable to move freely. The reason for this is that the muscles and blood vessels of the tongue are impaired, a condition which occurs, for example, during chronic disease (Fig. **44**). This patient suffers from lupus erythematosus with extreme weakness and generalized pain.

If the tongue is weak and flat, blood and *qi* (*xue qi*) are in a condition of deficiency. A dark, weak tongue is a sign that the body's *yin* is depleted. If the patient has recently fallen ill and has a dry, red, and weak tongue, this reveals that heat associated with the illness has burnt and damaged the *yin*.

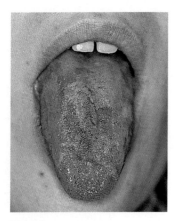

Fig. **44**

Systematic Procedure

2. The hard, stiff tongue

This tongue has lost its normal softness and elasticity and cannot therefore move freely. The cause can be found in an externally infectious heat disease, which has invaded deeply into the organism. Occasionally, this heat has penetrated into the pericardium, which corresponds to a typical syndrome of Chinese medicine. In addition, turbid phlegm (*tan*) may have blocked the interior of the body. This woman suffers from chronic hypertension (Fig. **45**).

However, it is also possible that severe heat has diminished the body fluids (Fig. **46**) and, therefore, a disturbing heat has had an especially strong influence on the organism. This kind of a tongue is frequently found in patients who are predisposed to a cerebral hemorrhage (stroke), but it can also occur in other disorders.

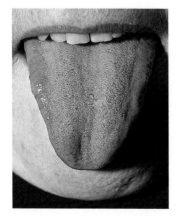

Fig. **45**

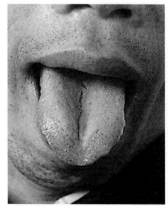

Fig. **46**

3. The slanting or oblique tongue

If the tongue hangs down on one side within the mouth, the patient has usually suffered a stroke, a cerebral hemorrhage (Fig. **47**, **48**).

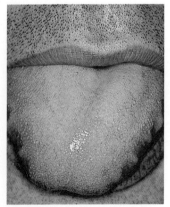

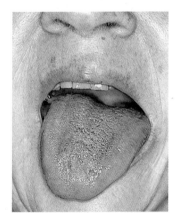

Fig. **47**

Fig. **48**

4. The shortened or shrunken tongue

A shortened tongue is always a sign of a serious, dangerous disease. If the tongue is at the same time light and moist or has a greenish color, it indicates a case of a cold stiffening of the muscles, vessels, and tendons (Fig. **49**).

A swollen and simultaneously shrunken tongue indicates that mucous and dampness have accumulated inside the organism. A pink, dry, and shrunken tongue suggests impairment of body fluids (*jin ye*) by a heat disease (Fig. **50**).

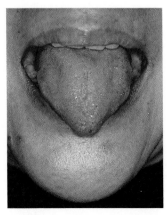

Fig. **49**

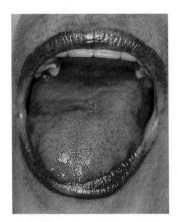

Fig. **50**

5. The trembling tongue

If a patient suffering from a long-standing illness shows a tongue which continuously trembles or vibrates, Chinese medicine refers to this as a "trembling tongue." It usually occurs in patients whose blood circulation (*xue qi*) is deficient or where there may be a severe deficiency of *yang* functions (*yang qi*). It can also signify heat disorder where severe heat has generated internal wind, which Chinese medicine refers to as "liver wind blows inside the organism."

6. The restless, protruding tongue

If the tongue constantly licks the upper or lower lips or the corners of the mouth and the tip protrudes slightly, this is referred to in Chinese medicine as a "restless, protruding tongue." It is a sign of a heat condition in the heart and spleen. The protruding tongue alone is a sign of an attack of mucus (phlegm) on the heart with mental disorder, a disturbance of the *shen*. Such a tongue can likewise signify a disturbance of the body's resistance in general. In children the restless tongue can also be a symptom of an impending fit or epileptic seizure. Furthermore, it may indicate a retarded mental capacity (a weakness of the *jing shen*).

The Coating of the Tongue

The Color of the Coating

Criteria
- ■ White
- ■ Yellow, brown
- ■ Gray, black

A white coating is the most common. Any other discoloration of the tongue coating can be considered as further pathological development of the original white coating.

1. The white coating

This suggests a superficial syndrome (*biao*) together with a cold syndrome, for example in cases of the common cold (influenza) (Fig. **51**). If the white coating is dry, cracked, or powdery, this is indicative of an abundant heat disturbance inside the body which has impaired the body fluids (*jin ye*) (Fig. **52**). A powdery coating alone indicates the presence of summer heat and dampness, which has stagnated in the organism, thus causing a disturbance within the body.

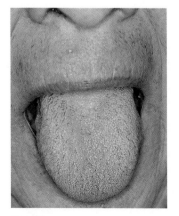
Fig. **51**

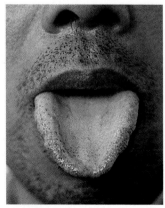
Fig. **52**

A white furred tongue can also appear at the beginning of an infectious disease (Fig. **53**), indicating an accumulation of pus or the presence of abscesses in the interior of the body.

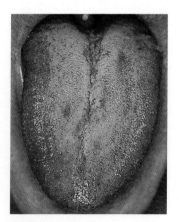

Fig. **53**

2. Yellow or brownish coating

This corresponds to an internal disease and to a heat syndrome. The darker the color, the more severe is the heat disturbance within the body. A light yellow color indicates slight heat (Fig. **54a**), whereas a dark yellow–coated tongue indicates severe heat, and a smoky yellow to brownish tongue reveals a stagnated heat disturbance deep inside the organism. If the body of the tongue is light, swollen, and soft, this indicates a *yang* deficiency with moistness and heat having accumulated internally (Fig. **54b**).

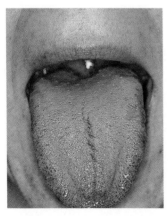

Fig. **54a**

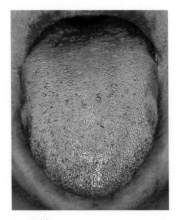

Fig. **54b**

3. The ash-gray or black coating

Both usually correspond to a heat syndrome, but can also be a sign of a cold wetness syndrome or a deficiency cold syndrome. Generally, this coating is only seen in patients who are seriously ill (Fig. **55**). Figure **56** shows the same patient, who suffered from a stroke and was half-paralyzed, after successful therapy with acupuncture and herbal prescriptions. The black discoloration has turned into a light brownish one.

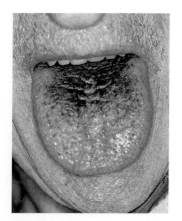

Fig. **55**

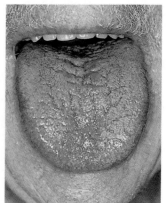

Fig. **56**

If the coating is ash-gray or black and dry, it suggests an impairment of the *yin* caused by burning heat. If the body of the tongue is light purple and the coating ash-gray or black and moist, this is an indication of a *yang* deficiency with abundant cold (Fig. **57**).

An ash-gray or black and moist coating is occasionally found in patients with phlegm (*tan yin*) accumulation and chest congestion who, however, are not seriously ill. This type of tongue must be clearly differentiated from the ash-gray and dark coating found in seriously ill patients.

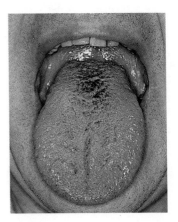

Fig. **57**

The Character and the Consistency of the Coating

Criteria

- Thin versus thick
- Moist versus dry
- Loose versus sticky (firmly adherent)
- Empty patches ("map tongue")
- Missing (complete absence of) coating

1. The thin versus thick coating

A thin coating is characteristic of slight or superficial disorders (Fig. **58**). It is often associated with infectious diseases which have not yet penetrated further into the body. If the coating is thick, it usually means that the disturbance has penetrated from the outside (*biao*) to the inside (*li*), or that stagnation has taken place within the body. If a person's condition deteriorates, a thin coating can develop further into a thick one. With a change for the better a thick coating gets thinner again. Figure **59** in addition shows a slight bluish discoloration of the body of the tongue, which is typical for blood stagnation.

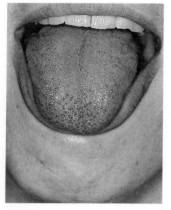

Fig. **58**

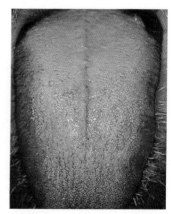

Fig. **59**

Systematic Procedure

2. The moist versus dry coating

A moist tongue coating reveals that the body fluids (*jin ye*) are not yet damaged (Fig. **60**). A furred tongue which is so watery that it "drips water," so to speak, to the extent that when the tongue protrudes the liquid runs down the tongue, suggests standing water within the body (Fig. **61**, **62**).

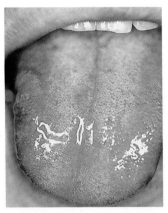

Fig. **60**

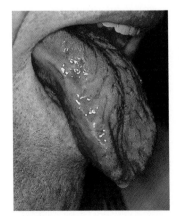

Fig. **61**

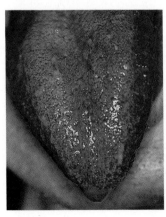

Fig. **62**

A totally dry coating, on the other hand, means complete absence of body fluids (Fig. **63**). It can also mean an external, infectious heat disease causing the dryness, whereby heat has damaged the body fluids. Or, alternatively, it can be the sign of a mixed disease with a *yin* deficiency and absence of saliva (Fig. **64**).

Another reason for a dry tongue could be that blood and *qi* fail to develop any fluid and that consequently the tongue looks dry.

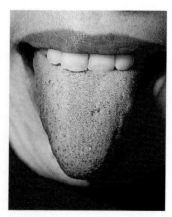

Fig. **63**

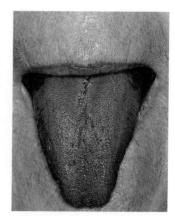

Fig. **64**

3. The loose versus sticky coating

The loose coating of the tongue, which lies lightly, loosely, and in large flakes on the surface of the tongue, is a sign of heat abundance and reveals that undigested food lies heavily in the stomach (Fig. **65**). This relates to a disturbance of the middle burner.

A sticky coating which cannot be scratched off consisting of fine flakes which are more numerous in the middle of the tongue, is a sign that there is a profuse mucous wetness within the body (Fig. **66**). Such a condition often results from wrong eating habits and is frequently found in adipose patients in European countries.

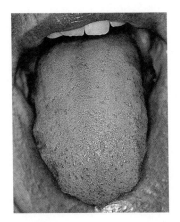

Fig. **65**

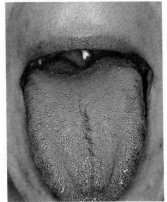

Fig. **66**

4. Empty patches on the tongue ("map tongue")

This refers to a tongue which is partly coated and partially without coating, so giving the tongue the appearance of a "map." The areas without coating look silky. This type of tongue indicates that there is insufficient *yin* in the stomach function. Such an appearance of the tongue reveals an emptiness of the liver *yin* if it shows up on the margin (Fig. **67**), or a deficiency of the stomach *yin* if it is seen in the middle of the tongue (Fig. **68**).

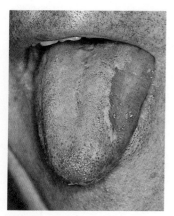

Fig. **67**

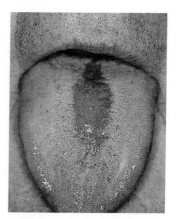

Fig. **68**

If the coating is sticky and firmly adhesive, it suggests that mucous wetness cannot be transformed inside the organism, or that the patient's resistance is impaired (Fig. **69**). In this case, the illness is quite serious.

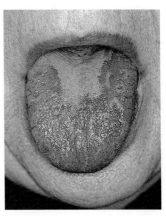

Fig. **69**

5. Missing (complete absence of) a coating

This is a sign that there is a lack of stomach *qi*, or it reveals an emptiness of the intestines and the kidney (lower burner). This elderly lady, for instance, suffers from diverticulitis and from chronic cystopyelitis (Fig. **70**).

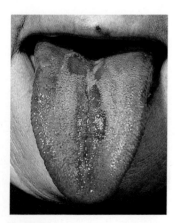

Fig. **70**

6. Observation of the course of a disease by evaluating the coating

If the normal coating gradually returns in time, it can be assumed that the stomach *qi* has recovered. If, in the case of an illness, no coating is initially visible, but then suddenly appears, this indicates either the development or the improvement of a stomach disorder. It can also indicate an acute attack of disturbing heat. If the patient has a coating on his or her tongue at the beginning of an illness which then suddenly disappears, it can be assumed that a serious weakness of stomach *qi* is present which is seriously threatening the basic life processes (Fig. **71**).

If a thick tongue coating gradually diminishes to a thin white coating, this indicates that the disturbance (*xie qi*) is gradually leaving the body and that the patient's condition is improving (Fig. **72a–d**). The consistency of a coating determines whether a disturbance is severe or slight. A wet or dry tongue indicates whether or not there are sufficient body liquids present. A loose or sticky coating is indicative of the amount of wetness or phlegm (mucus) or a weakness in the stomach and spleen. The appearance or disappearance of the coating of the furred tongue indicates that an illness is becoming worse or receding, respectively.

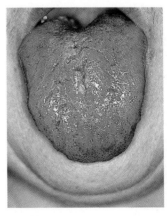

Fig. **71**

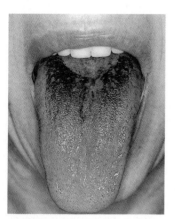

Fig. **72a**

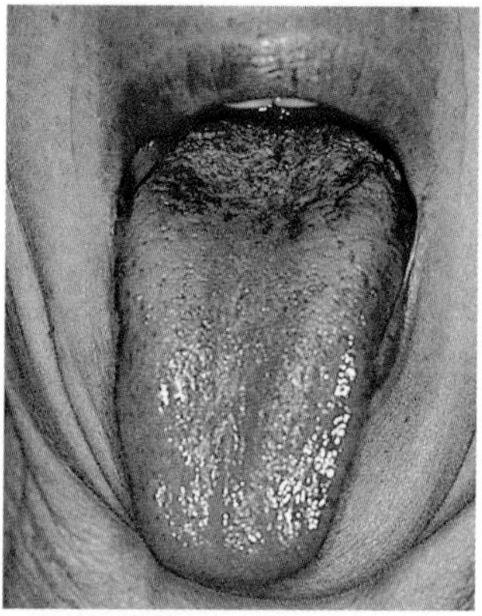

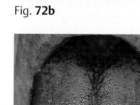

Fig. **72b**

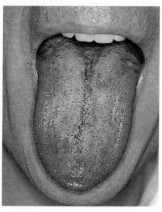

Fig. **72c**

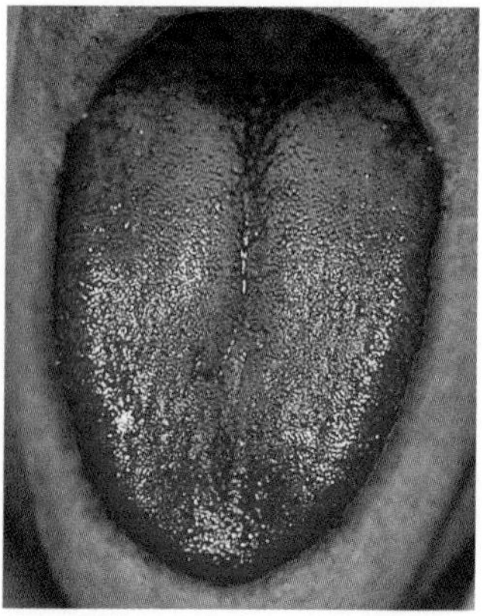

Fig. **72d**

Summary

In tongue diagnosis the Chinese physician observes changes in the
■ Body of the tongue,
■ Its consistency, and
■ Its coating.

Everything the physician observes in connection with the tongue
is collected and compared in order to produce a clear analysis of
the disease. The four diagnostic methods of
■ Viewing,
■ Hearing and smelling,
■ Taking the patient's history, and
■ Palpation (pulse diagnosis)

have to be employed jointly. The logical evaluation of all diagnostic features is finally summarized as the Differentiating Syndrome Diagnosis (*bian zheng*) of the individual patient, which
forms the basis for an effective treatment using acupuncture,
moxibustion, herbal prescription, or trophotherapy.

Clinical Part

Suggestions for Therapy

Recognition, Diagnosis, and Treatment

▶ Chapters 5–8

5 Clinical Applications

Preliminary Remarks

This chapter connects the various images of tongues that were systematically analyzed in Chapter 4 with suggestions for treatment by means of acupuncture, herbal prescription, and dietary measures (trophotherapy).

It goes without saying that the therapeutic suggestions given in the following are never to be employed in a stereotyped way. A proper Chinese therapy is always patient-centered, in other words, the whole individual human being must be taken into account before selecting the foramina (points), needles, herbs, or a dietary program.

Acupuncture requires a sound knowledge of special treatment rules and a high standard of manual dexterity, something which has to be studied and practised with a master for years. Mastery of Chinese prescription demands thorough studies of the properties of the individual herbs, minerals, and animal products, together with a knowledge of the important classical prescriptions from the basic sources. In addition, every ancient Chinese prescription should be adjusted to the requirements of the present-day Western individual, whose bodily, mental, and cultural conditions are slightly different from those of the ancient (and modern) Chinese. The same applies to the dietary recommendations given in the text.

Please find further information regarding *Chen Chiu* foramina, Chinese herbs (prescriptions), and dietetic recommendations as indicated below:

Chen Chiu Foramina

The syndrome effects of acupuncture foramina mentioned in this text can be found in Schnorrenberger, c.c.: Die topographisch- anatomischen Grundlagen der chinesischen Akupunktur und Ohrakupunktur, 6th ed. Stuttgart: Hippokrates Verlag (Bibliographical References 20) (1992).

Chinese Herbs (Prescription)

see. p. 293: List of Chinese Materia Medica

Dietetic Treatment

see. p. 283: Food Groups According to the Five Elements

Abbreviations used for acupuncture vessels (channels or meridians) and foramina (points) follow the WHO code of 1989:

Lung vessel	**LU**
Large intestine vessel	**LI**
Stomach vessel	**ST**
Spleen vessel	**SP**
Heart vessel	**HT**
Small intestine vessel	**SI**
Bladder vessel	**BL**
Kidney vessel	**KI**
Pericardium vessel	**PC**
Triple burner vessel	**TB**
Gallbladder vessel	**GB**
Liver vessel	**LR**
Governor vessel (*du mai*)	**GV**
Conception vessel (*ren mai*)	**CV**

The Light White Tongue

Fig. **73**: The color of this tongue is definitely lighter than normal. It corresponds to a cold and deficiency condition, which is usually a sign of weakness of the *yang* function (*yang qi*) and an insufficient blood supply of the organism.

Therapy According to Syndrome Differentiation

Strengthen *yang* and open up the surface

Chen Chiu Foramina

- ST-36
- CV (*ren mai*)-4, CV-6 (moxa!)
- LI-4

- KI-7
- BL-20, BL-23 (moxa!)
- GV (*du mai*)-20

- BL-15
- SP-10

Chinese Herbs (Prescription)

Use a variation of the Cinnamon Soup (first prescription from the *Shang Han Lun*) consisting of: *Cinnamomum cassia, Zingiber officinale, Ziziphus jujuba,* and *Glycyrrhiza uralensis.*

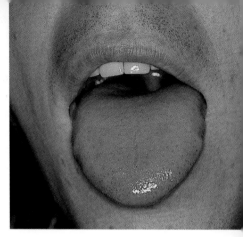

Fig. **73:** ▷ Color of the tongue body

Dietetic Treatment

- **To be avoided**

Avoid food with cold character (rhubarb, tropical fruits, watermelon, yogurt), frozen and uncooked food, ice-cream.

- **Recommended diet**

Eat warm meals and warm food from the earth and metal elements, for example leek, fennel, pumpkin, paprika. Taste: sweet, pungent. The sweet taste moistens; the pungent taste opens up the surface.

The Red Tongue (1)

Fig. **74**: This tongue is bright red and overall noticeably darker than a normal tongue. Such an appearance of the tongue corresponds to a heat condition and is usually a sign of an internal heat fullness syndrome. It can also be a sign of a *yin* deficiency associated with ascending internal fire (*xu huo*).

Therapy According to Syndrome Differentiation

Strengthen *yin*, cool heat

Chen Chiu Foramina

- SP-6
- CV (*ren mai*)-4
- GV (*du mai*)-14
- KI-3
- LI-4
- BL-40
- BL-23
- LI-11

Chinese Herbs (Prescription)

Rhemannia glutinosa, Poria cocos, Dioscorea batatas, Paeonia suffruticosa, Alisma plantago-aquatica, Cornus officinalis (Prescription: liu wei di huang wan).

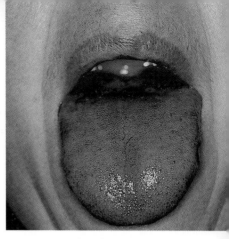

Fig. **74**: ▷ Color of the tongue body

Dietetic Treatment

- **To be avoided**

Avoid dood with hot and desiccating properties, especially hot alcoholic drinks, grilled meat, and bitter–hot spices.

- **Recommended diet**

Eat cold and refreshing meals from the wood element, for example all products made of soured milk, tomato, pineapple, and rhubarb, and those from the earth element, for instance cucumber, banana, mango, watermelon, and vegetables like broccoli, cauliflower, and eggplant.

The Red Tongue (2)

Fig. **75**: This tongue is red and noticeably darker than a normal tongue. Such a tongue corresponds to a pronounced internal heat condition and is usually a sign of an internal heat fullness syndrome. In this case, the internal heat is associated with wetness on the level of liver and gallbladder. This patient suffers from severe chronic hepatitis.

Therapy According to Syndrome Differentiation

Cool heat, excrete wetness, strengthen *yin*

Chen Chiu Foramina

- SP-6
- BL-25
- LI-11
- LR-2
- GV (*du mai*)-14
- BL-23
- LI-4

Chinese Herbs (Prescription)

Rhemannia glutinosa, Ophiopogon japonicus, Ziziphus jujuba (red dates), *Gypsum* (CaSO$_4$), *Nelumbo nucifera, Coptis chinensis, Lonicera japonica, Glycyrrhiza uralensis.*

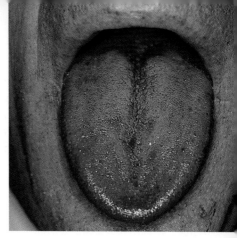

Fig. **75**: ▷ Color of the tongue body

Dietetic Treatment

- **To be avoided**

Avoid food with hot and desiccating properties, especially strong alcoholic drinks, grilled meat, and bitter–hot spices.

- **Recommended diet**

Eat cold and refreshing meals from the wood element, for example all products made of soured milk, tomato, pineapple, and rhubarb; and from the earth element, for instance cucumber, banana, mango, watermelon, and vegetables like broccoli, cauliflower, and eggplant.

The Dark Red Tongue

Fig. **76**: This tongue denotes a case of infectious heat disease whereby a heat disturbance has caused the pathological condition of a *ying fen* or *xue fen* syndrome.

If this type of tongue appears in a patient who is chronically ill, it indicates a *yin* deficiency with extreme fire. The deeper the color of the red or dark red tongue, the stronger the influence of the pathological heat disturbance. In this patient, a former drug addict, a central crease runs as far as the tip of the tongue, splitting it up into two halves, which indicates a serious disorder of the heart and the *shen* (cf. Fig. **24**).

Therapy According to Syndrome Differentiation

> **Strengthen *yin*, expel heat, and calm the heart**

Chen Chiu Foramina

- SP-6
- BL-23, BL-15, BL-14
- HT-3, HT-7

- KI- 3
- CV (*ren mai*)-4, CV-14
- GV (*du mai*)-14

- LI-2
- LR-11

Chinese Herbs (Prescription)

Rhemannia glutinosa and *fermentata (sheng di, shu di), Poria cocos, Ziziphus jujuba* (red dates), *Trichosanthes kirilowii, Ophiopogon japonicus, Asparagus cochinchinensis, Angelica sinensis, Paeonia lactiflora.*

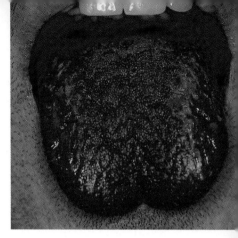

Fig. **76**:   ▷ Color and shape
of the tongue body

Dietetic Treatment

- **To be avoided**

Avoid especially hot food from the fire element such as hot spices, alcoholic drinks (whiskey, cognac), coffee, grilled meat, and food from the earth element with a hot character (e. g., fennel, cinnamon) in addition to food from the metal element, such as chillies, pepper, strong alcoholics (schnapps and brandy).

- **Recommended diet**

Eat cold and refreshing food (yogurt, buttermilk, green salad, fruit, and tropical fruit). Eat refreshing food from the fire element like artichoke, chicory, and dandelion (with a bitter taste). Drink enough liquid.

The Bluish-Green and the Purple Tongue

This tongue is of a greenish-purple color as a whole or displays purple or greenish spots on its surface. If the greenish-purple color is noticeably dark and the tongue is dry or just slightly moist, this is a pronounced heat effect. The purple tongue indicates blood stagnation (*yu xue*).

Fig. **77**: I treated this Chinese patient in 1977 at the *Hua-Dong* Hospital in Shanghai. The young woman suffered from a thrombocytopenia, which led to multiple bleeding into her joints (hemarthrosis) entailing severe joint pain. Chinese medicine refers to this condition as blood stagnation.

Fig. **78**: If the blue-purple discoloration is dark and the tongue is dry, this reveals an influence of internal heat after an external exposure to wind and cold. The patient shown is a Shanghai dock worker whom I saw and treated in 1977. He then suffered from acute bronchopneumonia.

Therapy According to Syndrome Differentiation

Dissolve blood stagnation

Fig. 78 in addition: Expel lung heat and dissolve phlegm

Chen Chiu Foramina

Fig. **77**:
- LI-4, LI-11
- CV (*ren mai*)-12
- SP-10
- BL-17, BL-20 (in addition to local foramina on the joints)

Fig. **78**:
- In addition to the above: LU-1, LU-7
- BL-12, BL-13

Chinese Herbs (Prescription)

Fig. **77**: *Carthamus tinctorius, Curcuma aromatica, Glechoma longituba, Prunus persica, Poria cocos, Dioscorea batatas, Angelica sinensis, Atractylodes macrocephala.*

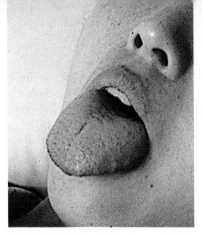
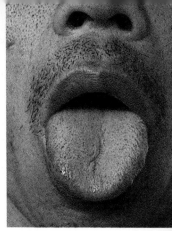

Fig. **77**: ▷ Color of the tongue body

Fig. **78**: ▷ Color of the tongue body

Fig. **78**: *Ephedra sinica, Astragalus membranaceus, Dioscorea bata-tas, Curcuma aromatica, Pinellia ternata, Trichosanthes kirilowii, Poria cocos, Glycyrrhiza uralensis.*

Dietetic Treatment

- **To be avoided**
Avoid food with warm and hot properties from the fire element that desiccate the system, for example coffee. Food with hot prop-erties from the metal element like chillies, curry, drinks like whiskey or Indian yogi tea.

- **Recommended diet**
Eat food with a refreshing character from the metal element (ef-fect on lung and intestines), for example, radish, cress, kohlrabi, mint. It is important to drink sufficient amounts of liquid (two or three liters daily). Recommended drinks: water, mint tea.

The Purple Tongue (2)

Fig. **79**: If the color of the purple tongue is lighter and it is moist, this suggests an influence of cold with blockage of blood and *qi*. Altogether the purple tongue is an important sign of blood stagnation (*yu xue*). The yellow spots in Figure **79** denote blocked internal heat in the organism.

Therapy According to Syndrome Differentiation

Dissolve blood blockage and excrete wetness

Expel cold and cool internal heat

Chen Chiu Foramina

- SP-6, SP-9, SP-10
- LI-4, LI-11
- CV(*ren mai*)-6, CV-12
- BL-17, BL-20, BL-23

Chinese Herbs (Prescription)

Carthamus tinctorius, Curcuma zedoaria, Dioscorea batatas, Atractylodes macrocephala, Angelica sinenesis, Poria cocos, Alisma plantago aquatica.

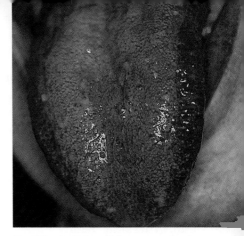

Fig. **79**: ▷ Color of the tongue body;
color and consistency
of the coating

Dietetic Treatment

- **To be avoided**

Avoid food with a refreshing and cool character, and food from the earth element with very sweet taste that humidifies the system.

- **Recommended diet**

Eat food with warm properties and metal-related food, for example onions, leeks, or red radishes. Eat food from the fire element like goat's cheese, oregano; drink cocoa and coffee.

The Wrinkled, Rough Tongue

Fig. **80**: The wrinkled, rough tongue with numerous grooves is called an "old" (*lao*) tongue. It corresponds to a fullness syndrome or a heat syndrome, or a diminished essence (*jing*) and is frequently seen in older people.

Fig. **81**: The wrinkled tongue shown presents numerous reddened foliate papillae on its tip as a sign of fire in the upper burner, in this case the heart; the patient suffers from mild insomnia and nervousness. The sticky yellow coating on the root signals a blockage of phlegm in the lower burner.

Therapy According to Syndrome Differentiation

> **Generate body liquids, cool heat; strengthen *yin*, support essence (*jing*)**

Chen Chiu Foramina

- LI-4, LI-11
- BL-23, BL-25
- CV (*ren mai*)-4, CV-12
- ST-36
- KI-3, KI-7

Fig. **81** in addition:
- SP-6, ST-40, HT-7

Chinese Herbs (Prescription)

Panax Ginseng, Codonopsis pilulosa, Astragalus membranaceus, Rhemannia glutinosa, Bupleurum chinense, Zizphus jujuba, (red dates), *Glycyrrhiza uralensis.*

Fig. **81** in addition: *Trichosanthes kirilowii, Poria cocos.*

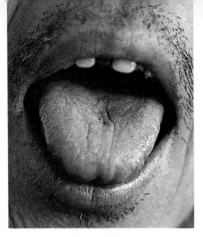

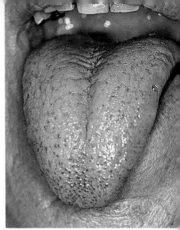

Fig. **80**: ▷ Shape of the tongue body

Fig. **81**: ▷ Shape of the tongue body

Dietetic Treatment

- **To be avoided**

Avoid food with hot and bitter taste from the metal and fire elements like onions and chillies.

- **Recommended diet**

Eat food with neutral and refreshing properties, a limited amount of cold food, and food from the earth and wood elements. Taste: sweet and sour. Drink enough liquid.

The Tender and Fine Tongue

Fig. **82**: Such a tongue is referred to as a "young" (*nen*) tongue; it indicates a mild deficiency and cold condition. The tongue shown is more or less still normal; it shows just a mild *yang* deficiency and a slight influence of cold.

Therapy According to Syndrome Differentiation

> Replenish emptiness,
> expel cold, and strengthen *yang*

Chen Chiu Foramina

- ST-36
- BL-15, BL-20, BL-23
- CV-6
- KI-7
- PC-6

Chinese Herbs (Prescription)

Angelica sinensis, Dioscorea batatas, Atractylodes macrocephala, Glycyrrhiza uralensis, Ziziphua jujuba (red dates).

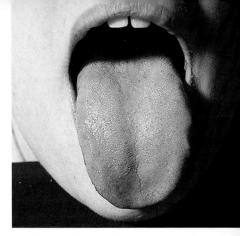

Fig. **82:** ▷ Shape of the tongue body

Dietetic Treatment

- **To be avoided**

Avoid food with a cold and refreshing character, frozen food (including ice-cream), uncooked food, tropical fruit, and yogurt (especially in the cold season).

- **Recommended diet**

Eat food with a warm character from the earth element. Taste: sweet and pungent. Eat walnuts to reinforce *yang*.

The Swollen Tongue (1)

Fig. **83**: This tongue is larger and thicker than a normal tongue. If the color of the swollen tongue is light and white, this is a sign of an emptiness of the *qi* and *yang* in the spleen and stomach.

Fig. **84**: This female patient, in addition, presents tooth marks on both sides of her tongue, which is typical for a *yang* deficiency. There is a sticky coating indicating an accumulation of mucus (phlegm) in the middle and the lower burner.

Therapy According to Syndrome Differentiation

Replenish *qi* and *yang*; strengthen the spleen and the stomach

Chen Chiu Foramina

- ST-36
- BL-20, BL-23

- CV-4, CV-6 (moxa)
- CV-12

Fig. **84** in addition:
- SP-6, SP-10, ST-40

Chinese Herbs (Prescription)

Zingiber officinalis, Dioscorea batatas, Atractylodes macrocephala, Astragalus membranaceus, Codonopsis pilulosa, Glycyrrhizas uralensis, Panax Ginseng, Cinnamomum cassia, Poria cocos.

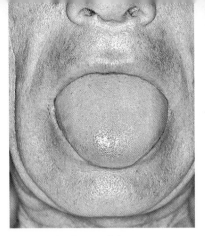
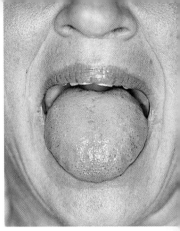

Fig. **83:** ▷ Shape of the tongue body

Fig. **84:** ▷ Shape of the tongue body

Fig. **84**: *Leave Panax Ginseng out! Instead: Angelica sinensis, Pinellia ternata.*

Dietetic Treatment

- **To be avoided**

Avoid food with cold and refreshing properties from the wood element with sour taste, milk products.

- **Recommended diet**

Eat warm and hot dishes from the earth element (e. g., fennel, cinnamon, potato, pumpkin). Eat warm meals and roasted cereals.

The Swollen and Red Tongue (2)

Fig. **85**: If the swollen tongue is red, it shows that there is an internal heat or a profuse disturbing heat (in Chinese medicine called "poisonous" heat) with a deficiency of *yin* inside the organism. The tooth marks reveal a simultaneous *yang* deficiency.

Therapy According to Syndrome Differentiation

> **Replenish *yin*, cool and excrete heat, and strengthen *yang***

Chen Chiu Foramina

- SP-6
- ST-36
- KI-3
- BL-23, BL-15
- GV (*du mai*)-14
- CV (*ren mai*)-4

Chinese Herbs (Prescription)

Ophiopogon japonicus, Asparagus cochinchinensis, Ziziphus jujuba (red dates), *Angelica sinensis, Rhemannia glutinosa, Trichosanthes kirilowii, Glycyrrhiza uralensis.*

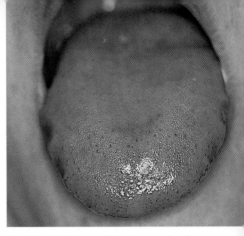

Fig. **85**: ▷ Shape of the tongue body

Dietetic Treatment

- **To be avoided**

Avoid food with too hot or too cold properties and food from the fire element.

- **Recommended diet**

Eat cereals with a sweet taste (e. g., wheat, barley, buckwheat, millet), soy sprouts; cereals with a salty taste (black rice, *Zizania palustris*); refreshing uncooked food, as well as milk products; watermelon and cucumber.

The Thin, Small Tongue

Fig. **86**: A thin, small tongue which is light in color usually indicates a deficiency of blood and *qi* (*xue qi*) or it reveals that both heart and spleen are in a condition of emptiness. Such a condition can often be found in young intellectuals (college or university students) with psychosomatic disorder such as lack of appetite, insomnia, forgetfulness, nervousness, and palpitations.

Therapy According to Syndrome Differentiation

> **Replenish blood and *qi*, and strengthen spleen and heart**

Chen Chiu Foramina

- ST-36
- CV-4, CV-6, CV-12
- BL-23, BL-20, BL-15
- SP-6, SP-10
- KI-7
- HT-7

Chinese Herbs (Prescription)

Panax Ginseng, Dioscorea batatas, Ziziphus jujuba, Glycyrrhiza uralensis, Poria cocos, Atractylodes macrocephala, Codonopsis pilulosa, Rhemannia glutinosa, Cinnamomum cassia.

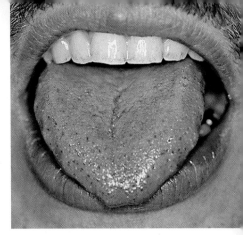

Fig. **86**: ▷ Shape of the tongue body

Dietetic Treatment

- **To be avoided**

Avoid bitter foods that desiccate the organism (strong coffee, red wine, spirits), and too rich and too greasy meals.

- **Recommended diet**

Eat humidifying food from the earth element with a sweet taste, for example fennel and paprika. Serve food from the wood element (with a sour taste), for example tomatoes.

The Dark Red, Thin, and Small Tongue

Fig. **87**: A dark red, thin, small tongue corresponds to a *yin* emptiness with an abundance of heat, rendering the body fluids (*jin ye*) diminished or impaired. This is usually a sign of a serious disease. The patient depicted here is a rather tall man but his tongue is not at all in proportion with his body height. He suffers from high blood pressure, insomnia, and diabetes due to *yin* deficiency and internal heat, which has diminished his body liquids.

Therapy According to Syndrome Differentiation

Replenish *yin* and expel heat

Chen Chiu Foramina

- SP-6
- KI-3, KI-7
- BL-23, BL-25
- GV (*du mai*)-14
- CV (*ren mai*)-4
- LI-4, LI-11

Chinese Herbs (Prescription)

Angelica sinensis, Ophiopogon japonicus, Asparagus cochinchinensis, Rhemannia fermentata (shu di), Glycyrrhiza uralensis, Anemarrhena asphodeloides, Pueraria lobata, Rhemannia glutinosa (sheng di).

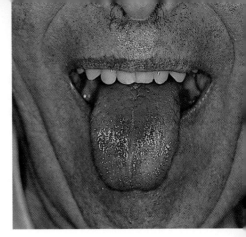

Fig. **87**: ▷ Color and shape
of the tongue body

Dietetic Treatment

- **To be avoided**

Avoid food with a pungent and bitter taste, food with hot properties from the fire and the metal elements (grilled meat, bitter liqueurs, pepper).

- **Recommended diet**

Eat neutral and refreshing food, a limited amount of food with cold properties, and green vegetables. Drink sufficient amounts of liquid (two or three liters daily).

The Fissured Tongue

Fig. **88**, **89**: If the tongue has many transverse and longitudinal fissures with cracks and grooves in it, it is referred to as a "fissured tongue." If such a tongue is also dark red, this usually shows an abundance of heat. The patient in Figure **88** suffers from a severe and generalized allergy.

If such a tongue is white and light in appearance, this can indicate a lack of *yin* and blood. The patient shown in Figure **89** suffers from multiple disorders of his gastrointestinal tract, including hepatitis in his history.

Therapy According to Syndrome Differentiation

Replenish *yin*, strengthen blood, and expel heat

Chen Chiu Foramina

- SP-6
- ST-36
- BL-23, BL-12
- LR-2 or LR-3
- CV (*ren mai*)-4, CV-12
- GV (*du mai*)-14
- SP-10
- LI-4, LI-11

Chinese Herbs (Prescription)

Angelica sinensis, Ophiopogon japonicus, Trichosanthes kirilowii, Bupleurum chinense, Asparagus cochinchinensis, Glycyyrrhiza uralensis, Rhemannia fermentata (shu di).

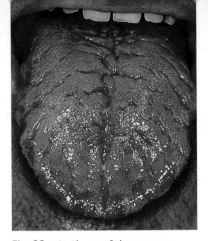

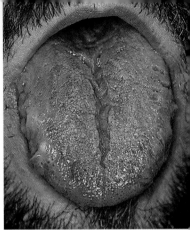

Fig. **88**: ▷ Shape of the tongue body

Fig. **89**: ▷ Shape of the tongue body

Dietetic Treatment

- **To be avoided**

Avoid pungent and bitter food from the metal and fire elements, food with warm and hot properties, for example coffee, red wine, goat's cheese, grilled meat, chillies, Indian yogi tea.

- **Recommended diet**

Eat food with neutral and refreshing properties; consume a limited amount of cold dishes. Taste: sweet, slightly sour, and salty.

The Tongue With "Tooth Marks"

Fig. **90**: Tooth marks on both edges of the tongue are usually found in a swollen tongue. The teeth press against the tongue because it has become too large for the oral cavity. It is especially patients suffering from a deficiency of the *yang qi* who present this.

Such a tongue can develop rapidly, in cases of severe exhaustion even within a few hours. After the person recovers, such a tongue can quickly return to normal.

Therapy According to Syndrome Differentiation

Replenish *yang* and strengthening *qi*

Chen Chiu Foramina

- ST-36 (moxa)
- BL-20, BL-15
- BL-23 (moxa)
- CV (*ren mai*)-6 (moxa)
- HT-5
- CV (*ren mai*)-12

Chinese Herbs (Prescription)

Cervus nippon, Panax Ginseng, Dioscorea batatas, Atractylodes macrocephala, Poria cocos, Angelica sinensis, Zingiber officinalis (dried root), *Glycyrrhiza uralensis, Cinnamomum cassia.*

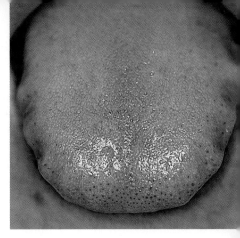

Fig. **90:** ▷ Shape of the tongue body

Dietetic Treatment

- **To be avoided**

Avoid frozen and uncooked food, tropical fruit in wintertime, cold food from the wood element.

- **Recommended diet**

Eat neutral and warming food, walnuts to reinforce the *yang*, and sweet food (e.g., wholemeal bread) from the earth element, and pungent food (mustard) from the metal element.

The Granular Tongue (Granular Papillae 1)

Fig. **91**: Such a tongue appears when the filiform papillae get larger and thicker than normal, or when they transform into fungiform papillae. A granular tongue suggests a profuse, severe external heat disturbance. The more intense the external heat, the larger the red granules on the tongue become. If these appear on the tip of the tongue, this is a sign of abundant heart–fire (cf. Fig. **41 and 92**). If the granules are located on the sides of the tongue, this is an indication of abundant fire in the liver and gall bladder (cf. Fig. **42 and 93 a, b**). If they show up in the middle of the tongue, this is a sign of an abundant heat in the spleen, stomach, and intestines. The more the granular papillae move toward the tip of the tongue, the more severe is the involvement of the upper burner (heart, lungs, pericardium) (cf. Fig. **43 and 94**).

Therapy According to Syndrome Differentiation

Cool heat, calm the heart, and dissolve phlegm (mucus)

Chen Chiu Foramina

- GV (*du mai*)-14
- KI-3
- SP-6

- CV (*ren mai*)-4, -14
- LI-11
- BL-23, BL-15

- HT-3, HT-7

Chinese Herbs (Prescription)

Bupleurum chinense, Pinellia ternata, Poria cocos, Paeonia lactiflora, Glycyrrhiza uralensis, Rhemannia glutinosa, Ophiopogon japonicus, Citrus aurantium.

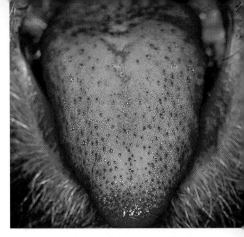

Fig. 91: ▷ Shape of the tongue body

Dietetic Treatment

- **To be avoided**

Avoid a bitter and pungent taste from the fire and metal elements; hot and warm dishes.

- **Recommended diet**

Chinese green tea, watermelon, drink at least two or three liters daily. Eat cold, refreshing, and neutral food from the wood and earth elements (pears, tropical fruit, etc.).

Granular Papillae (2)

Fig. **92**: If the granular papillae appear on the tip of the tongue, this is a sign of abundant heart–fire.

Therapy According to Syndrome Differentiation

> **Strengthen *yin*, cool heat, excrete fire, and calm the heart**

Chen Chiu Foramina

- SP-6
- HT-3, HT-7
- CV (*ren mai*)-6
- BL-15, BL-23

Chinese Herbs (Prescription)

Gardenia jasminoides, Rhemannia glutinosa, Coptis chinensis, Ziziphus jujuba, Glycyrrhiza uralensis, Ophiopogon japonicus.

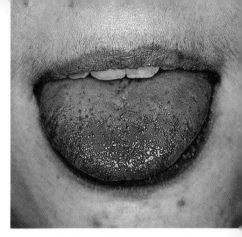

Fig. **92**: ▷ Shape of the tongue body

Dietetic Treatment

- **To be avoided**

Avoid hot and warm food from the fire element like coffee, cocoa, spirits, red wine, and grilled meat. Serve hot and warm food from the metal element, for example onions and garlic.

- **Recommended diet**

Drink sufficient water (two or three liters daily); eat watermelon with neutral and refreshing food from the wood element (spelt), and from the earth element (corn, cauliflower, broccoli).

Granular Papillae (3)

Fig. **93a**: If the granules are located on the edges of the tongue, this is an indication of abundant fire in the liver and gallbladder.

Therapy According to Syndrome Differentiation

Cool heat, calm the liver, and strengthen *yin*

Chen Chiu Foramina

- LR-2, LR-3, LR-14
- GV (*du mai*)-14
- SP-6
- BL-18, BL-23

Chinese Herbs (Prescription)

Paeonia lactiflora, Bupleurum chinense, Fritillaria cirrhosa, Allium macrostemon, Poria cocos, Glycyrrhiza uralensis, Angelica sinensis, and *Ophiopogon japonicus.*

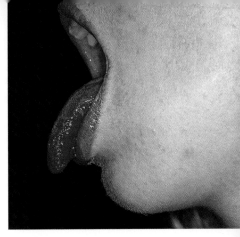

Fig. **93a**:   ▷ Shape of the tongue body

Dietetic Treatment

- **To be avoided**

Avoid hot and warm food from the fire element like coffee, cocoa, spirits, red wine, and grilled meat.

- **Recommended diet**

Drink sufficient amounts of water (two or three liters daily), eat watermelon and refreshing and cold food from the wood element (buttermilk, yogurt, sauerkraut, tomatoes, and pineapple).

Granular Papillae (4)

Fig. **93b**: If the granules show up in the middle of the tongue, this is a sign of an abundant heat in the spleen, stomach, and intestines (middle burner).

Therapy According to Syndrome Differentiation

Cool heat, strengthen the middle burner, nourish and replenish *yin*

Chen Chiu Foramina

- ST-44, ST-37, ST-25
- CV-12
- BL-20, BL-23, BL-25
- LI-4, LI-11

Chinese Herbs (Prescription)

Gardenia jasminoides, Poria cocos, Ziziphus jujuba (red dates), *Ophiopogon japonicus, Glycyrrhiza uralensis, Angelica sinensis, Paeonia lactiflora.*

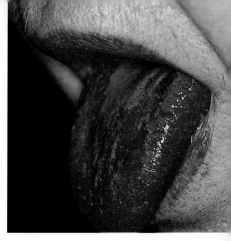

Fig. **93b**: ▷ Shape of the tongue body

Dietetic Treatment

- **To be avoided**

Avoid hot and warm food from the fire element such as coffee, cocoa, spirits, red wine, and grilled meat.

- **Recommended diet**

Drink sufficient water (two or three liters daily). Eat watermelon and neutral, refreshing food from the earth element (e. g., millet, corn, cabbage).

Granular Papillae (5) on the Tip

Fig. **94**: The more the granular papillae move toward the tip of the tongue, the more severe is the involvement of the **upper burner** (heart, lungs, pericardium).

Therapy According to Syndrome Differentiation

> **Cool heat, excrete fire, calm the heart, and replenish *yin***

Chen Chiu Foramina

- SP-6
- HT-3

- CV (*ren mai*)-4
- BL-15, BL-23
- GV (*du mai*)-14

Chinese Herbs (Prescription)

Gardenia jasminoides, Rhemannia glutinosa, Coptis chinensis, Poria cocos, Ziziphus jujuba, Ophiopogon japonicus, Glycyrrhiza uralensis.

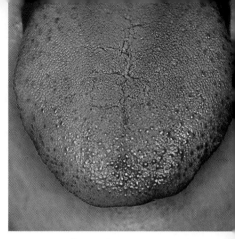

Fig. **94**: ▷ Shape of the tongue body

Dietetic Treatment

- **To be avoided**

Avoid hot and warm food from the fire element such as coffee, cocoa, spirits, as well as red wine and grilled meat.

- **Recommended diet**

Drink sufficient water (two or three liters daily). Eat watermelon and food from the cold group of the fire element, and drink Chinese green tea. Eat food from the fire element with refreshing properties, like artichoke, and food from the metal element which nourishes the lung (onions, garlic, red radish, radish, cress).

The Weak, Frail Tongue

Fig. **95**: This tongue is weak and without force. It is unable to move freely. The reason is that the muscles and blood vessels of the tongue are impaired, a condition which occurs, for example, during severe chronic disease. This patient suffers from lupus erythematosus with extreme weakness of the body and generalized pain. If the tongue is weak and flat, blood and *qi* (*xue qi*) are in a condition of deficiency.

A dark, weak tongue is a sign that the patient's essence (*jing*) and the body's *yin* are depleted. If the patient has recently fallen ill and has a dry, red, and weak tongue, according to Chinese medicine this reveals that heat associated with his or her illness has "burnt" the *yin*.

Therapy According to Syndrome Differentiation

> **Strengthen blood and *yin*, strengthen the spleen, strengthen the kidney, and dissolve phlegm (mucus)**

Chen Chiu Foramina

- SP-6
- LI-11, LI-4
- BL-23, BL-20
- ST-36, ST-40
- PC-6
- CV (*ren mai*)-6
- GV (*du mai*)-14

Chinese Herbs (Prescription)

Angelica sinensis, Panax Ginseng, Paeonia lactiflora, Pinellia ternata, Atractylodes macrocephala, Dioscorea batatas, Rhemannia glutinosa, and *Glycyrrhiza uralensis.*

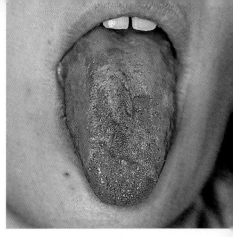

Fig. **95**:   ▷ Consistency of the tongue

Dietetic Treatment

- **To be avoided**

Avoid hot and warm food from the fire and metal elements and sweet food that produces phlegm.

- **Recommended diet**

Eat chicken soup with Angelica root, food from the water element (seafood, lobster), and cold food from the fire element like dandelion leaves. Furthermore, consume food from the earth element that strengthens the spleen (corn, pumpkin). Recommended drinks: Chinese green tea, fresh water (two or three liters daily).

The Hard, Rigid Tongue (1)

Fig. **96**: This tongue has lost its normal softness and elasticity and cannot therefore move freely. The cause can be found in an externally infectious heat disease which has invaded deeply into the organism. Occasionally, this heat has penetrated into the pericardium, which corresponds to a typical syndrome of Chinese medicine. In addition, turbid phlegm (*tan*) may have blocked the interior of the body. This woman suffers from chronic (essential) hypertension and mental depression; some years ago she had her gallbladder removed because of cholelithiasis (gallstones).

Therapy According to Syndrome Differentiation

Cool heat, dissolve phlegm (mucus), calm the liver, and excrete wetness

Chen Chiu Foramina

- SP-6, SP-9
- PC-3, PC-6
- BL-18
- GV (*du mai*)-14
- ST-40
- BL-20, BL-23
- LR-3, LR-14

Chinese Herbs (Prescription)

Paeonia lactiflora, Pinellia ternata, Anemarrhena asphodeloides, Poria cocos, Grifola umbellata, Bupleurum chinense, Ostrea gigas, Coix lachrymajobi, and *Glycyrrhiza uralensis.*

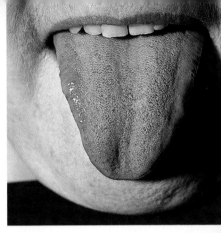

Fig. **96**: ▷ Consistency of the tongue

Dietetic Treatment

- **To be avoided**

Avoid food with hot properties, very sour food with astringent properties that retains liquids, humidity, and phlegm within the organism.

- **Recommended diet**

Eat warm food from the metal element, for example onions, leek, garlic with a pungent taste and dissolving character, and food with warm properties from the fire element, for example cheese made from sheep's milk, poppy seeds, oregano. For eliminating humidity and phlegm use different kinds of beans. Add *Coix lachryma-jobi* (cf. herbal prescription above) to the dishes.

The Hard, Stiff Tongue (2)

Fig. **97**: It is also possible that severe heat has diminished the body fluids (*jin ye*) and, therefore, a disturbing heat has had an especially strong influence on the organism as shown here. The patient worked in a political cadre of the local Communist party in Shanghai when I saw him at the *Hua-Dong* Hospital in 1977 and was, like many people in mainland China in those days, a chain smoker. He complained of chronic bronchitis, insomnia and bouts of headache. In addition to the marked rigidity of his tongue, a generalized sticky gray–yellow coating associated with numerous reddened foliate papillae on the tip is visible. This kind of hard, stiff tongue is frequently found among patients who are predisposed to a cerebral hemorrhage (stroke) (cf. the special case of a hard, stiff tongue depicted in Fig. **99**), but it can also occur in association with other disorders.

Therapy According to Syndrome Differentiation

> Dissolve phlegm (mucus), calm the liver, excrete wetness, and divert heat from the pericardium

Chen Chiu Foramina

- ST-36, ST-40
- SP-6, SP-9
- BL-14, BL-23, BL-25
- PC-6, PC-7
- LR-3, LR-14
- LU-1, LU-7

Chinese Herbs (Prescription)

Pinellia ternata, Bupleurum chinense, Paeonia lactiflora, Coix lachrymajobi, Gardenia jasminoides, Ziziphus jujuba, Poria cocos, Glycyrrhiza uralensis.

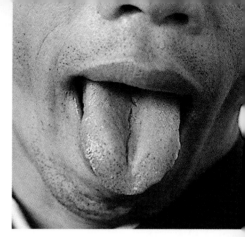

Fig. **97**: ▷ Consistency of the tongue

Dietetic Treatment

- **To be avoided**

Avoid food with hot properties and very sour food because of its astringent effect (fixation of humidity and phlegm in the organism).

- **Recommended diet**

Eat warm food from the metal element, for example onions, leek, garlic with hot taste and dissolving character, and food with warm properties from the fire element, for example cheese made from sheep's milk, poppy seeds, oregano. For eliminating humidity and phlegm use different kinds of beans. Add boiled *Coix lachrymajobi* to the dishes.

The Slanting or Oblique Tongue

If the tongue hangs down on one side within the mouth, the patient has usually suffered a stroke, a cerebral hemorrhage.

Fig. **98**: A mild case of cerebral hemorrhage in a younger male (slightly slanting tongue).

Fig. **99**: Pronounced case of a slanting, oblique tongue. Strong internal heat has diminished the body liquids, causing an even more dangerous internal heat or fire, which according to Chinese medicine results in "internal wind" (*zhong feng*) leading to a stroke with hemiplegia. This case is a special form of hard, stiff tongue (cf. Fig. **97**).

Therapy According to Syndrome Differentiation

Calm the liver, expel liver (internal) wind, strengthen the kidney *yin*, clam the *shen*, strengthen the spleen

Chen Chiu Foramina

- LI-4, LI-11
- GB-20
- GV (*du mai*)-14, GV-20

- BL-15, BL-18, BL-23
- LR-3, LR-14
- CV (*ren mai*)-6, CV-12

- AP-3 (*yin tang*)

Chinese Herbs (Prescription)

Bupleurum chinensis, Paeonia lactiflora, Ostrea gigas, Haliotis diversicolor, Hematite, Stegodon orientalis, Rhemannia glutinosa, Ophiopogon japonicus, and *Glycyrrhiza uralensis.*

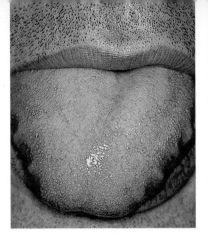
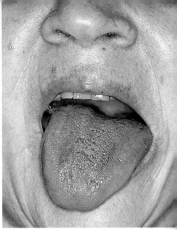

Fig. **98**: ▷ Consistency
of the tongue

Fig. **99**: ▷ Consistency
of the tongue

Dietetic Treatment

- **To be avoided**

Avoid hot food from the fire element, for example coffee, schnapps, and grilled meat. Do not use too pungent food from the metal element.

- **Recommended diet**

Eat warm and neutral food from the earth element, for example celery, carrots, and refreshing food from the wood element such as tomatoes, cucumber, pickled gherkins. The kidney *yin* can be strengthened with squid (cuttlefish) and chicken meat.

The Trembling Tongue

The trembling tongue usually occurs in patients whose blood circulation (*xue qi*) is deficient or where there may be a severe deficiency of *yang* functions (*yang qi*). It can also signify an external heat disorder where severe heat has generated internal wind (*zhong feng*) which Chinese medicine refers to as "liver wind blows inside the organism."

Therapy According to Syndrome Differentiation

Calm the liver, expel liver wind, strengthen the spleen, and strengthen *qi* and *yang*

Chen Chiu Foramina

- SP-6, SP-10
- LI-4, LI-11
- ST-36
- GV (*du mai*)-14
- BL-18, BL-23
- GB-20
- LR-3

Chinese Herbs (Prescription)

Paeonia lactiflora, Bupleurum chinense, Ostrea gigas, Stegodon orientalis, Uncaria rhynchophylla, Atractylodes macrocephala, Ziziphus jujuba, Trichosanthes kirilowii, and *Glycyrrhiza uralensis.*

Dietetic Treatment

- **To be avoided**

Avoid hot food from the fire element, for example coffee, schnapps, grilled meat, and pungent food from the metal element.

- **Recommended diet**

Eat warm or neutral food from the earth element (potatoes, corn) and walnuts to reinforce *yang*. Use warm and neutral food from the metal element such as onions, leeks, and garlic.

The Shortened or Shrunken Tongue (1)

Fig. **100**: A shortened tongue is always a sign of a serious, dangerous disease. If the tongue is at the same time light and moist or has a greenish color, it indicates a case of a cold stiffening of the muscles, vessels, and tendons. This young Chinese woman living in London is an international business executive with a lot of professional stress and tension. When she came to see me she suffered from severe exhaustion (chronic fatigue syndrome) with numbness of parts of her skin, muscle weakness in her lower legs and low back pain. The consultants could not specify any neurological or internal disorder. She was treated with acupuncture, moxibustion, and Chinese herbs and her condition improved markedly within several months. After one year she had recovered completely.

Therapy According to Syndrome Differentiation

Strengthen *yin*, dissolve phlegm (mucus), expel heat, excrete wetness, and generate body liquids

Chen Chiu Foramina

Angelica sinensis, Curcuma zedoaria, Rhemannia glutinosa (sheng di), Paeonia lactiflora, Poria cocos, Grifola umbellata, Pinellia ternata, Dioscorea batatas, Atractylodes macrocephala.

Chinese Herbs (Prescription)

Rhemannia glutinosa, Paeonia lactiflora, Poria cocos, Alisma plantago-aquatica, Angelica sinensis, Pinellia ternata, Atractylodes macrocephala.

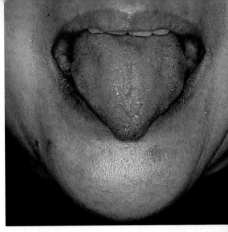

Fig. **100**: ▷ Consistency of the tongue

Dietetic Treatment

- **To be avoided**

Avoid hot food, very sour dishes because of their astringent properties that hold body liquids and humidity in the organism.

- **Recommended diet**

Eat warm food from the metal element, for example rice wine, onions, leeks (dissolving character, pungent taste). Use different kind of beans to eliminate humidity and phlegm.

The Shortened or Shrunken Tongue (2)

Fig. **101**: A swollen and simultaneously shrunken tongue indicates that phlegm (mucus) and dampness have accumulated inside the organism. Body fluids (*jin ye*) impaired by a heat disease cause a pink, dry, and shrunken tongue (cf. Fig. **100**).

Therapy According to Syndrome Differentiation

Cool heat, divert fire, and strengthen *yin* and blood

Chen Chiu Foramina

- SP-6
- LI-4, LI-11
- GB-20
- ST-36, ST-44
- BL-20, BL-23, BL-40
- KI-3
- GV (*du mai*)-14

Chinese Herbs (Prescription)

Gardenia jasminoides, Ophiopogon japonicus, Lilium brownii, Lycium barbarum, Angelica sinensis, Zizphus jujuba, Bupleurum chinense, Glycyrrhiza uralensis.

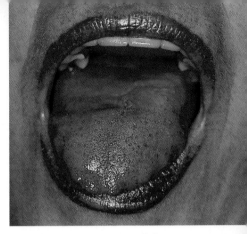

Fig. **101**: ▷ Consistency of the tongue

Dietetic Treatment

- **To be avoided**

Avoid hot food from the fire element, for example coffee, schnapps, grilled meat, black tea.

- **Recommended diet**

Eat refreshing and cold food from all five elements. Drink sufficient amounts of water (two or three liters daily) and Chinese green tea. Use asparagus to reinforce *yin*. Serve vegetable soup with *Angelica sinensis* to strengthen the blood (one liter of water plus two spoons of Angelica root, to be cooked for 30 minutes).

The Restless, Protruding Tongue

This is a sign of a heat condition in the heart and spleen. The protruding tongue alone is a sign of an attack of mucus (phlegm) on the heart with a mental disorder, a disturbance of the *shen*. Such a tongue can likewise signify a disturbance of the body's resistance in general. In children, the restless tongue can be a symptom of an impending fit or epileptic seizure. Furthermore, it may indicate a retarded mental capacity (a weakness of the *jing shen*).

Therapy According to Syndrome Differentiation

Calm heart and *shen*, calm the liver, excrete poisonous heat, and strengthen *yin*

Chen Chiu Foramina

- SP-6
- HT-3, HT-7
- GV (*du mai*)-14, GV-20
- ST-36
- LI-11
- BL-14, BL-15, BL-18, BL-23

Chinese Herbs (Prescription)

Stegodon orientalis, Paeonia lactiflora, Bupleurum chinense, Ostrea gigas, Gardenia jasminoides, Zizphus jujuba, Rhemannia glutinosa, Glycyrrhiza uralensis.

Dietetic Treatment

- **To be avoided**

Avoid hot food from the fire element (grilled meat, goat's milk, goat's cheese), alcoholic drinks, too spicy dishes.

- **Recommended diet**

Eat dandelion leaves and asparagus that nourish *yin*, and oysters to calm the liver. Recommended beverage: Chinese green tea.

The White Coating (1)

A white coating is the most common. All other discoloration of the tongue coating can be considered as the further pathological development of the original white coating.

Fig. **102**: This suggests a superficial (*biao*) syndrome together with a cold syndrome, for example in cases of common cold (influenza). Such a thin white coating is a typical sign of a *tai yang* disease as portrayed in the first chapter of the *Shang Han Lun*. The patient is a young Chinese schoolboy aged 11 whom I saw and treated in Hong Kong. If the white coating is dry, cracked, or powdery, it is indicative of an abundant heat disturbance inside the organism which has impaired the body fluids (*jin ye*) (cf. Fig. **103**).

Therapy According to Syndrome Differentiation

> **Loosen up the surface (*jie biao*) and expel the heat disturbance**

Chen Chiu Foramina

- LI-4, LI-11
- GV (*du mai*)-14
- GB-20
- BL-12, BL-13
- ST-36, ST-40
- CV (*ren mai*)-4

Chinese Herbs (Prescription)

The Cinnamon soup (first prescription of the *Shang Han Lun*) consisting of: *Cinnamomum cassia, Paeonia lactiflora, Glycyrrhiza uralensis, Zingiber officinalis, Ziziphus jujuba.*

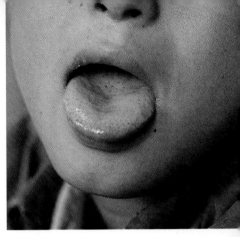

Fig. **102**: ▷ Color of the tongue coating

Dietetic Treatment

● **To be avoided**
Avoid hot food from the fire element (grilled meat, goat's milk and goat's cheese). Do not consume drinks such as coffee, black tea, espresso.

● **Recommended diet**
Eat neutral and refreshing food from the metal element. In case of a heat disturbance serve peppermint and soy beans (cf. List of Chinese Materia Medica, Group 1b, p. 289).

The White Coating (2)

Fig. **103**: A powdery coating alone indicates the presence of summer heat and dampness (wetness) which has stagnated in the organism, thus causing a disturbance within the body. A white furred tongue can also appear at the beginning of an infectious disease, indicating an accumulation of pus or the presence of abscesses inside the body. The figure shows the tongue of a Shanghai dock worker suffering from bronchopneumonia; in this case, phlegm (mucus) is also present.

Therapy According to Syndrome Differentiation

> **Open the lung and bronchi (*xuan fei*), open up the surface, and dissolve phlegm**

Chen Chiu Foramina

- LU-1, LU-7
- BL-12, BL-13, BL-23
- ST-36, ST-40
- GV (*du mai*)-14
- LI-11

Chinese Herbs (Prescription)

The Small Blue Dragon Soup (twenty-first prescription of the *Shang Han Lun*): Ephedra sinica, Paeonia lactiflora, Asarum heterotropoides, Zingiber officinale, Glycyrrhiza uralensis, Cinnamomum cassia, Schizandra chinensis, Pinellia ternata.

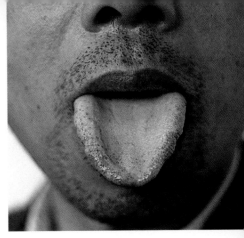

Fig. **103**:   ▷ Color of the tongue coating

Dietetic Treatment

- **To be avoided**

Avoid hot food from the fire element and milk products that generate phlegm and humidity.

- **Recommended diet**

Eat warm and refreshing food from the metal element, such as onions, horseradish, leeks, cress.

The White Coating (3)

A white furred tongue which appears at the beginning of an infectious disease indicates an accumulation of pus or the presence of abscesses inside the body.

Fig. **104a**: This is the tongue of a male patient suffering from hepatitis.

Fig. **104b**: This shows the tongue of a 50-year-old female patient with bronchiectasis.

Therapy According to Syndrome Differentiation

Fig. 104a: Calm and activate the liver, excrete poisonous heat–wetness	Fig. 104b: Open up the lung and bronchi, cool heat, and dissolve phlegm

Chen Chiu Foramina

- LI-4, 11, LR-3 (2), LR-14
- PC-6, BL-18, BL-19, ST-36
- CV (*ren mai*)-6, GV-14, GV-20
- NP-88 (gan yan)

- LU-1, LU-7, LI-4, LI-11
- BL-13, BL-23, ST-36, ST-40
- CV (*ren mai*)-6

Chinese Herbs (Prescription)

Paeonia lactiflora, Bupleurum chinense, Uncaria rhynchophylla, Trichosanthes kirilowii, Glycyrrhiza uralensis, Coptis chinensis, Scutellaria baicalensis.

Ephedra sinica, Pinellia ternata, Zingiber officinale, Astragalus membranaceus, Glycyrrhiza uralensis.

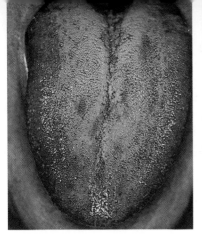

Fig. **104a**: ▷ Color of the tongue coating

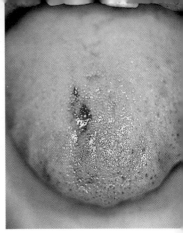

Fig. **104b**: ▷ Color of the tongue coating

Dietetic Treatment

- **To be avoided**

Avoid food from the fire element; hot food from the earth element.

Avoid too cold food, sweet-tasting food from the earth element; milk products that generate phlegm.

- **Recommended diet**

Cooking methods that nourish yin; food from the wood element with refreshing properties.

Eat food from the metal element, for example radish, mustard, cress.

The Yellow Coating (1)

Fig. **105**: This coating is a transformation of the white coating. It corresponds to an internal disease and to a heat syndrome. The darker the color, the more severe is the heat disturbance within the body. A light yellow color indicates slight heat, whereas a dark yellow–coated tongue indicates severe heat, and a smoky yellow to brownish tongue reveals a stagnated heat disturbance deep inside the organism (cf. Fig. **106**).

Therapy According to Syndrome Differentiation

> **Cool heat, divert fire, and replenish *yin***

Chen Chiu Foramina

- LI-4, LI-11
- GV (*du mai*)-14
- SP-6
- BL-20, BL-23

Chinese Herbs (Prescription)

Anamarrhena asphodeloides, Pueraria lobata, Bupleurum chinense, Paeonia lactiflora.

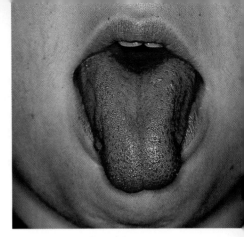

Fig. **105**: ▷ Color of the tongue coating

Dietetic Treatment

● **To be avoided**
Avoid hot food from all the five elements and do not use cooking methods that reinforce *yang*.

● **Recommended diet**
Eat refreshing food from the metal element, for example white radish and mustard, and asparagus that nourishes *yin*. Use cooking methods that strengthen *yin*.

The Yellow Coating (2)

Fig. **106**: If the body of the tongue with a yellow coating is light, swollen, and soft, this indicates a generalized *yang* deficiency with wetness and heat accumulated internally.

Therapy According to Syndrome Differentiation

Divert heat and fire, excrete wetness from the intestines, and strengthen the spleen

Chen Chiu Foramina

- GV (*du mai*)-14
- HT-3
- CV (*ren mai*)-12
- LI-11
- ST-25, ST-40
- BL-23
- SP-9

Chinese Herbs (Prescription)

Poria cocos, Grifola umbellata, Atractylodes macrocephala, Dioscorea batatas, Coptis chinensis, Scutellaria baicalensis, Glycyrrhiza uralensis.

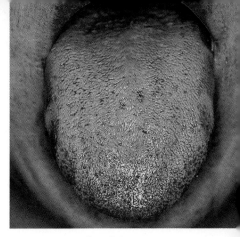

Fig. **106**:   ▷ Color of the tongue coating

Dietetic Treatment

● **To be avoided**
Avoid hot food from all five elements and use cooking methods that reinforce *yang*.

● **Recommended diet**
Eat warm and refreshing food from the metal element and asparagus to nourish *yin*. Use cooking methods that reinforce *yin*.

The Ash-Gray or Black Coating (1)

Fig. **107a**: Both usually correspond to a heat syndrome, but can also be a sign of a cold–wetness syndrome or a deficiency cold syndrome. Generally, this coating is only seen in patients who are seriously ill. The accumulation of internal heat has lead to a *zhong feng* syndrome in this patient who suffered from liver–fire and internal wind.

Fig. **107b**: The same patient, who after a cerebral hemorrhage was half-paralyzed and unable to walk around and to move his right arm and leg. Needle therapy and herbal prescription were successful. He was able to walk without a stick after 12 treatments and within four weeks. By that time, the black discoloration had turned into a light brownish one.

Therapy According to Syndrome Differentiation

Nourish *yin*, expel heat, calm the liver, and divert fire

Chen Chiu Foramina

- KI-3, KI-6
- ST-36
- BL-23, BL-25
- LI-4, LI-11
- CV (*ren mai*)-4 , CV-6
- SP-6
- GV (*du mai*)-14
- LR-2 (3)
- KI-6

Chinese Herbs (Prescription)

Paeonia lactiflora, Bupleurum chinense, Ostrea gigas, Haliotis diversicolor, Stegodon orientalis, Uncaria rhynchophylla, Glycyrrhiza uralensis, Ophiopogon japonicus, Gypsum ($CaSO_4$).

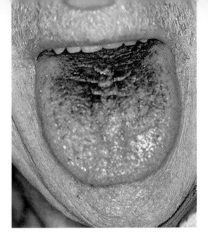

Fig. **107a**: ▷ Color of the tongue
coating

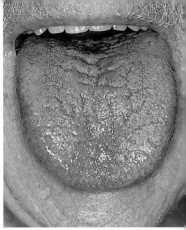

Fig. **107b**: ▷ Color of the tongue
coating

Dietetic Treatment

- **To be avoided**

Avoid hot food from all five elements and do not use cooking
methods that reinforce *yang* (grilling or pickling). Avoid beverages like alcohol and coffee.

- **Recommended diet**

Serve oysters to calm the liver in addition to warm and refresh-
ing food from the metal element. Eat asparagus to nourish *yin*.
Use cooking methods that reinforce *yin*. Recommended beverage:
Chinese green tea.

The Ash-Gray or Black Coating (2)

- If the coating is ash-gray or black and dry, this suggests an impairment of the *yin* by burning heat. The patient in Figure **108** suffers from chronic constipation and an adenoma of his prostate.
- If the body of the tongue is light purple and the coating ash-gray or black and moist, this is an indication of a *yang* deficiency with abundant cold.
- An ash-gray or black and moist coating is also found in patients with phlegm (*tan yin*) accumulation and chest congestion who, however, are not seriously ill.

This type of tongue must be clearly differentiated from the ash-gray and dark coating found in seriously ill patients as shown in Figure **107a**.

Therapy According to Syndrome Differentiation

> **Strengthen kidney *yin*, excrete poisonous heat, and dissolve phlegm**

Chen Chiu Foramina

- KI-3
- SP-6, SP-9
- CV (*ren mai*)-3, CV-6
- ST-36, ST-40
- LI-4, LI-11
- GV (*du mai*)-1, GV-14
- BL-23, BL-25
- LU-1

Chinese Herbs (Prescription)

Pinellia ternata, Dioscorea batatas, Astragalus membranaceus, Ziziphus jujuba, Glycyrrhiza uralensis, Angelica sinensis, Alisma plantago-aquatica, Scutellaria baicalensis.

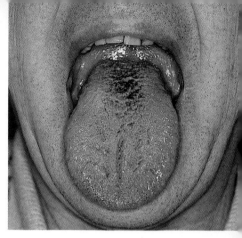

Fig. **108:** ▷ Color of the tongue coating

Dietetic Treatment

• **To be avoided**
Avoid hot and warm food and drinks from the fire element with desiccating properties (coffee, spirits, grilled meat).

• **Recommended diet**
Eat warm and refreshing food from the metal element that open up the surface and support the metabolism and the secretion of waste products. Reinforce kidney *yin* with seafood, carrots, and chicken meat. Recommended drinks: Chinese green tea plus sufficient amounts of water (two or three liters daily).

The Thin Coating

Fig. **109**: A thin coating is characteristic of slight disturbances or superficial disorders. It is often associated with infectious diseases which have not yet penetrated further into the body. Due to seasonal influences a thin coating is normally found in autumn.

Therapy According to Syndrome Differentiation

Loosen (open) up the surface and expel the exterior disturbance

Chen Chiu Foramina

- LI-4, LI-11
- ST-36, ST-40
- BL-15, BL-40
- GV (*du mai*)-14

Chinese Herbs (Prescription)

The Cinnamon Soup (*Shang Han Lun*) consisting of: *Cinnamomum cassia, Paeonia lactiflora, Glycyrrhiza uralensis, Zingiber officinalis, Ziziphus jujuba.*

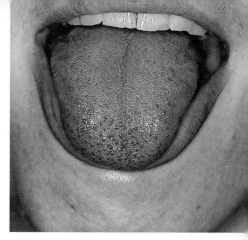

Fig. **109**: ▷ Character and consistency of the coating

Dietetic Treatment

- **To be avoided**

Avoid food from the fire element, like coffee, with a desiccating effect.

- **Recommended diet**

Eat hot and warm food from the metal element, for example onions, mustard, garlic, ginger, and red radish.

The Thick Coating

Fig. **110**: A thick coating usually indicates that the disturbance has penetrated from the outside (*biao*) to the inside (*li*), or that stagnation has taken place within the body. In this case, an accumulation of phlegm has invaded into all the three burners. As a disease develops, a thin coating can develop further into a thick one. With a change for the better a thick coating gets thinner again. Figure **110** in addition reveals a slight bluish discoloration of the body of the tongue, which is typical for blood stagnation (*yu xue*). The patient shown here is a heavy smoker, a salesman with irregular eating habits. He suffers from lower back pain and severe indigestion with constipation in addition to chronic bronchitis and attacks of stenocardia.

Therapy According to Syndrome Differentiation

> **Dissolve phlegm, dissolve blood blockage, and strengthen spleen and kidney**

Chen Chiu Foramina

- LI-11
- BL-14, BL-20, BL-23
- ST-36, ST-40
- CV (*ren mai*)-4, CV-12

Chinese Herbs (Prescription)

Pinellia ternata, Rhemannia glutinosa, Carthamus tinctorius, Atractylodes macrocephala, Astragalus membranaceus, Glycyrrhiza uralensis.

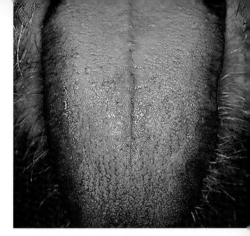

Fig. **110**: ▷ Character and consistency
of the coating

Dietetic Treatment

- **To be avoided**

Avoid food which is too cold or too refreshing. No greasy meals as they cause an accumulation of phlegm. Avoid very sweet food as it generates humidity and phlegm. No food produced by extraction methods such as flour, white sugar, and all kinds of sweets should be used.

- **Recommended diet**

Eat organic food from the earth element to strengthen the spleen. Serve dishes like seafood, chicken meat, walnuts, and leek to reinforce the kidneys.

The Moist Coating (1)

Fig. **111**: A moist tongue coating reveals that the body fluids (*jin ye*) are abundant.

Therapy According to Syndrome Differentiation

Strengthen the spleen, and excrete water and wetness

Chen Chiu Foramina

- LI-4, LI-11
- BL-20, BL-23
- ST-36
- LU-1
- CV (*ren mai*)-23

Chinese Herbs (Prescription)

Poria cocos, Grifola umbellata, Alisma plantago-aquatica, Atractylodes macrocephala, Pinellia ternata, Glycyrrhiza uralensis.

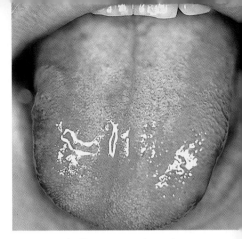

Fig. **111**: ▷ Character and consistency
of the coating

Dietetic Treatment

- **To be avoided**

Avoid too sweet food as it favors an accumulation of humidity, as well as too sour and astringent food that prevents body juices from being excreted.

- **Recommended diet**

Eat warm and neutral food from the earth element, for example pumpkin, potatoes, carrots, millet, and corn (to strengthen the spleen). Serve dishes from the metal element like curry powder, leeks, horseradish, mustard, cress.

The Very Moist or Watery Tongue

Fig. **112a**: A fissured tongue which is so watery that it "drips water" to the extent that when the tongue protrudes the liquid runs down the tongue suggests standing water within the organism.

Fig. **112b**: If the color is dark purple and the tongue is very wet, this indicates blood stagnation (*yu xue*) in addition to water accumulation in the body.

Therapy According to Syndrome Differentiation

Fig. 112a: Excrete water and wetness, strengthen the spleen	Fig. 112b: Excrete wetness, dissolve blood blockage, strengthen the spleen

Chen Chiu Foramina

- SP-6, SP-9, BL-20, BL-23
- CV (*ren mai*)-4, CV-12
- KI-7, LI-11

- LI-4, LI-11, BL-17, BL-20
- SP-10, BL-20, BL-23, ST-36
- CV (*ren mai*)-3, CV-12

Chinese Herbs (Prescription)

Poria cocos, Grifola umbellata, Alisma plantago-aquatica, Akebia trifoliata, Talcum, Atractylodes macrocephala, Glycyrrhiza uralensis.

Poria cocos, Grifola umbellata, Carthamus tinctorius, Curcuma aromatica, Atractylodes macrocephala, Glycyrrhiza uralensis.

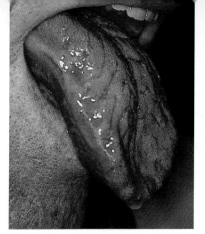
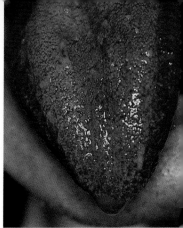

Fig. **112a**: ▷ Character and consistency of the coating

Fig. **112b**: ▷ Character and consistency of the coating

Dietetic Treatment

- **To be avoided**

Avoid sweet food, in particular refined (white) sugar.

- **Recommended diet**

Eat warm and neutral food from the earth element (organic products). Serve warm and neutral food from the metal element, for example onions, leeks, ginger.

The Dry Coating (1)

Fig. **113**: An absolutely dry coating indicates a complete absence of body fluids (cf. Fig. **63**). It can also indicate an external, infectious heat disease causing the dryness, whereby heat has damaged the body fluids. Or, alternatively, it can be the sign of a mixed disease with a *yin* deficiency and a lack of saliva (cf. Fig. **114**).

Therapy According to Syndrome Differentiation

Generate body liquids, strengthen the spleen, and dissolve phlegm (mucus

Chen Chiu Foramina

- LI-4, LI-11
- LU-1, LU-7
- ST-36, ST-40
- GV (*du mai*)-14
- BL-12, BL-13
- SP-6

Chinese Herbs (Prescription)

Pinellia ternata, Poria cocos, Grifola umbellata, Glycyrrhiza uralensis, Astragalus membranaceus, Ephedra sinica.

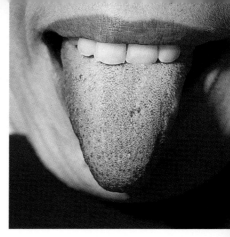

Fig. **113**:   ▷ Character and consistency
of the coating

Dietetic Treatment

- **To be avoided**
Avoid desiccating food from the fire element and drinks like coffee, spirits, and red wine.

- **Recommended diet**
Eat sweet food from the earth element; asparagus as it nourishes *yin*. Serve warm and refreshing food from the metal element to open up the surface (lung).

The Dry Coating (2)

Fig. **114**: Another reason for a dry coating is a deficiency of blood and *qi* resulting in a retarded production of body liquids. Therefore, the coating looks dry as in this elderly female patient who is suffering from a weakness of her essence (*jing*) and *yin*.

Therapy According to Syndrome Differentiation

Nourish *yin*, invigorate blood, and strengthen the spleen

Chen Chiu Foramina

- SP-6
- BL-20, BL-23
- CV (*ren mai*)-4, CV-6, CV-12
- KI-3
- LI-11

Chinese Herbs (Prescription)

Ophiopogon japonicus, Asparagus cochinchinensis, Equus asinus, Rhemannia fermentata (shu di), Angelica sinensis, Atractylodes macrocephala, Glycyrrhiza uralensis.

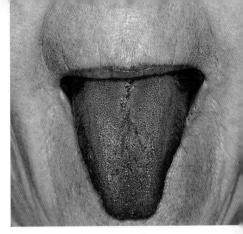

Fig. **114**:   ▷ Character and consistency
of the coating

Dietetic Treatment

- **To be avoided**

Avoid cooking methods that reinforce *yang* (grilling, pickling, roasting, very hot dishes) and food from the fire element. Drinks: no coffee, red wine, and spirits (brandy, schnapps).

- **Recommended diet**

Eat food from the earth element. Use cooking methods that reinforce *yin*. Serve vegetable soup containing Angelica root (one liter of water, two spoons of Angelica, to be cooked for 30 minutes).

The Loose Coating

Fig. **115**: The loose coating of the tongue, which lies lightly, loosely, and in large flakes on the tongue's surface, is a sign of abundant heat and reveals that undigested food lies heavily in the stomach (cf. Fig. **65**). This condition is related to a disturbance of the middle burner.

Therapy According to Syndrome Differentiation

Cool heat, control fire, and dissolve phlegm (mucus)

Chen Chiu Foramina

- ST-36, ST-40
- LI-4, LI-11
- BL-20
- CV (*ren mai*)-12

Chinese Herbs (Prescription)

Trichosanthes kirilowii, Gardenia jasminoides, Pinellia ternata, Citrus aurantium, Atractylodes macrocephala, and *Glycyrrhiza uralensis.*

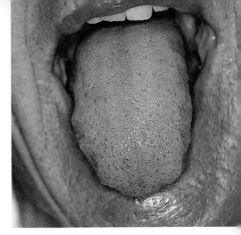

Fig. **115**: ▷ Character and consistency of the coating

Dietetic Treatment

- **To be avoided**

Avoid hot food from the fire element with a heating character. No uncooked food that impairs the digestive functions. Avoid very sweet food as it supports the production of phlegm.

- **Recommended diet**

Eat warm or neutral food from the earth element and cooked cereals. Recommended drinks: Chinese green tea, fresh water.

The Sticky Coating

Fig. **116**: A sticky coating which cannot be scratched off and consisting of numerous fine flakes in the middle of the tongue is a sign of a profuse mucous wetness associated with phlegm in the body. Such a condition often results from wrong eating habits and is frequently found in obese Europeans. Figure **116**, in addition, reveals a slight yellow tinge of the coating indicating heat.

Therapy According to Syndrome Differentiation

Dissolve phlegm (mucus) and excrete wetness–heat

Chen Chiu Foramina

- ST-40
- SP-6, SP-9
- BL-15, BL-20
- LI-11
- CV (*ren mai*)-12
- GV (*du mai*)-14

Chinese Herbs (Prescription)

Pinellia ternata, Trichosanthes kirilowii, Astragalus membranaceus, Ziziphus jujuba, Glycyrrhiza uralensis, Scutellaria baicalensis.

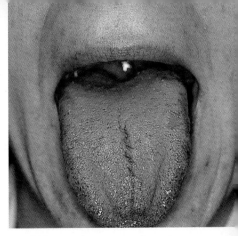

Fig. **116**:   ▷ Character and consistency
of the coating

Dietetic Treatment

- **To be avoided**

Avoid hot food from the fire element and uncooked food that impairs digestive functions and very sweet food that supports the production of phlegm.

- **Recommended diet**

Eat warm and neutral food from the earth element in addition to cooked cereals. Recommended drinks: Chinese green tea, fresh water.

Empty Patches on the Tongue ("Map Tongue") (1)

Fig. **117:** This refers to a tongue which is partly coated and partially without coating, so giving the tongue the appearance of a "map." The areas without coating look smooth and silky. This type of a tongue indicates that there is insufficient *yin* in the liver or in the stomach function. If such an appearance of the tongue shows up on the margin it reveals an emptiness of the liver *yin*.

If the coating is sticky and firmly adhesive, it suggests that mucous wetness cannot be transformed inside the organism, or that the patient's resistance is impaired (cf. Figs. **118–120**). In such cases, the illness is quite serious.

Therapy According to Syndrome Differentiation

Calm the liver and strengthen stomach *yin*

Chen Chiu Foramina

- SP-6
- ST-20, ST-21, ST-36, ST-40
- LI-4, LI-11 (cf. Fig. **117**, **119**)
- LR-3, LR-14
- BL-18, BL-20, BL-23

Chinese Herbs (Prescription)

Paeonia lactiflora, Gallus gallus domesticus, Oryza sativa, Ophiopogon japonicus, Haliotis diversicolor, Ostrea gigas, and Glycyrrhiza uralensis.

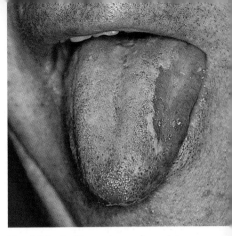

Fig. **117:** ▷ Character and consistency
of the coating

Dietetic Treatment

- **To be avoided**

Avoid hot and desiccating food from the fire element, alcohol, hot
spices, and greasy meals.

- **Recommended diet**

A medical check-up for an possible lack of vitamins is recommended. Eat food from the earth element, and warm and neutral
food from the metal element, oysters that calm the liver. Use cooking methods that reinforce *yin.*

Empty Patches on the Tongue ("Map Tongue") (2)

Fig. **118**: The specific location of the empty patches on the tongue will indicate which corresponding interior organs have to be strengthened. This tongue reveals a disturbance of the middle and lower burners (deficiency of stomach *yin*, spleen *qi*, kidney and bladder) with an accumulation of wetness and phlegm which cannot be excreted (cf. Figs. **117**, **119**).

Therapy According to Syndrome Differentiation

> **Strengthen the spleen and stomach *yin*, strengthen the lower burner (kidneys), dissolve phlegm (mucus)**

Chen Chiu Foramina

- SP-6
- ST-20, ST-21, ST-36, ST-40
- LI-4, LI-11
- LR-3, LR-14
- BL-18, BL-20, BL-23

Chinese Herbs (Prescription)

Rhemannia glutinosa, Paeonia lactiflora, Poria cocos, Dioscorea batatas, Pinellia ternata, Glycyrrhiza uralensis.

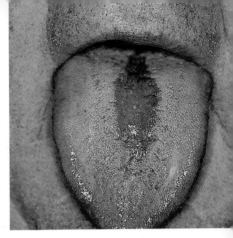

Fig. **118**: ▷ Character and consistency
of the coating

Dietetic Treatment

- **To be avoided**

Avoid hot and desiccating food from the fire element. No cooking
methods that reinforce *yang*.

- **Recommended diet**

Eat food from the water element, for example seafood, algae, and
sushi. Serve food from the metal element (horseradish) that opens
up the surface of the system and eliminates humidity.

Empty Patches on the Tongue ("Map Tongue") (3)

Fig. **119**: If the coating is sticky and firmly adhesive, it suggests that mucous wetness cannot be transformed inside the organism and cannot be excreted, or it reveals that the patient's resistance is impaired (cf. Fig. **69**). In this case, there is phlegm associated with wetness–heat within the lower burner; the missing coating in the middle and on the margin of the tongue indicates a weakness of the middle burner and an impairment of the liver.

Therapy According to Syndrome Differentiation

> Excrete wetness–heat from the lower burner, nourish *yin*, strengthen the spleen, and calm the liver

Chen Chiu Foramina

- SP-6
- ST-20, ST-21, ST-36, ST-40
- LI-4, LI-11
- LR-3, LR-14
- BL-18, BL-20, BL-23

Chinese Herbs (Prescription)

Angelica sinensis, Rhemannia glutinosa, Atractylodes macrocephala, Paeonia lactiflora, Anemarrhena asphodeloides, Coptis chinensis, Bupleurum chinensis, Glycyrrhiza uralensis, Pinellia ternata.

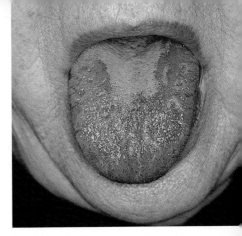

Fig. **119**: ▷ Character and consistency
of the coating

Dietetic Treatment

- **To be avoided**
Avoid hot food from the fire element. Do not use cooking methods that reinforce yang.

- **Recommended diet**
Eat food from the water element, for example seafood, algae, and sushi. Serve food from the metal element (horseradish) that opens up the surface and eliminates humidity.

The Missing Coating

Fig. **120**: This is a sign that there is a lack of stomach *qi* or it reveals a weakness of the intestines and an emptiness of the kidney (lower burner). This elderly woman, for instance, suffers from a diverticulitis and from chronic cystopyelitis. If the normal coating gradually returns, it can be assumed that the stomach *qi* and the disturbance of the intestines have recovered (cf. Figs. **121–125**).

Therapy According to Syndrome Differentiation

Strengthen kidney *yin*, direct off internal heat and fire, generate body liquids

Chen Chiu Foramina

- BL-20, BL-23
- ST-36, ST-37
- SP-6
- KI-3
- CV (*ren mai*)-4

Chinese Herbs (Prescription)

Paeonia lactiflora, Rhemannia glutinosa, Angelica sinensis, Ziziphus jujuba, Dioscorea batatas, Glycyrrhiza uralensis.

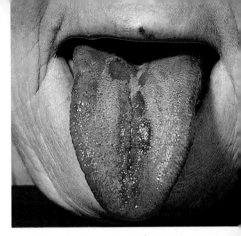

Fig. **120:** ▷ Character and consistency
of the coating

Dietetic Treatment

- **To be avoided**

Avoid hot food from the fire element. Do not use cooking methods that reinforce *yang*. No hot spices. Avoid beverages like red
wine, brandy, and coffee.

- **Recommended diet**

Eat food from the earth element (dairy products) and from the
water element (seafood). Serve warm and neutral food from the
metal element. Drink sufficient water (two or three liters daily)
and Chinese green tea.

The Missing and Black Coating (1)

Fig. **121**: This patient suffers from severe chronic pain of her thoracic and lumbar spine for which she was successfully treated with acupuncture. This photograph was taken following a relapse three years after the first treatment. Her tongue shows a black discoloration in addition to a missing coating on the root (lower burner). This reveals an emptiness of the kidneys related to the sore lumbar region. It should be remembered that according to Chinese medicine most cases of chronic lower back pain including herniated disks are symptomatic of either kidney *yin* or *yang* emptiness (cf. Fig. **122**).

Therapy According to Syndrome Differentiation

Nourish the kidney *yin*, dissolve phlegm, and excrete internal heat

Chen Chiu Foramina

- BL-15, BL-23, BL-25, BL-40, BL-52
- ST-36, ST-40
- KI-7
- SP-6
- GV (*du mai*)-3

Chinese Herbs (Prescription)

Rhemannia glutinosa, Alisma plantago-aquatica, Angelica sinensis, Cornus officinalis, Dioscorea batatas, Glycyrrhiza uralensis.

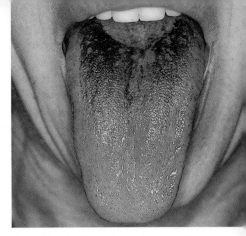

Fig. **121**: ▷ Character and color of the coating

Dietetic Treatment

- **To be avoided**

Avoid hot and desiccating food from the fire element. Do not use cooking methods that reinforce *yang* and hot spices. Hazardous drinks: red wine, brandy, and coffee.

- **Recommended diet**

Eat food from the earth and water elements, for example seafood. Serve warm to neutral dishes from the metal element. Recommended beverages: Drink enough water (two or three liters daily) and Chinese green tea.

The Missing and Black Coating (2)

Fig. **122**: After five treatment sessions with acupuncture the black coating has turned into a white-yellowish one. This shows an improvement of the internal heat condition. In conjunction with this, the pain in the spinal column has subsided and the prognosis is favorable.

Therapy According to Syndrome Differentiation

Nourish the kidney *yin*, dissolve phlegm, and excrete internal heat

Chen Chiu Foramina

- BL-15, BL-23, BL-25, BL-40, BL-52
- ST-36, ST-40
- KI-7
- SP-6
- GV (*du mai*)-3

Chinese Herbs (Prescription)

Rhemannia glutinosa, Alisma plantago-aquatica, Angelica sinensis, Cornus officinalis, Dioscorea batatas, Glycyrrhiza uralensis.

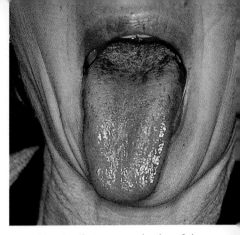

Fig. **122**:   ▷ Character and color of the coating

Dietetic Treatment

- **To be avoided**

Avoid food from the fire element as well as hot spices. Do not use cooking methods that reinforce *yang*. Beverages: red wine, brandy, and coffee should be avoided.

- **Recommended diet**

Eat food from the earth element (millet) and from the water element (seafood), warm food from the metal element (leek, cheese made from cow's milk, chives). Recommended beverages: Two or three liters of water daily; Chinese green tea to eliminate the heat.

The Missing and White Coating

Fig. **123**: A white coating on a markedly red tongue body. The margin of this tongue is especially red and without coating around the edges, an appearance related to a liver disease. This patient suffers from a severe nonA, nonB hepatitis (cf. Fig. **124**). The differentiating syndrome diagnosis (*bian zheng*) here is "wetness and heat in liver and gallbladder."

Therapy According to Syndrome Differentiation

> **Calm and support the liver (*shu gan*), excrete wetness–heat from liver and gallbladder**

Chen Chiu Foramina

- LR-2 (or LR-3), LR-14
- SP-6, SP-9
- BL-18, BL-19, BL-23
- GB-24
- NP (new point)-88 (*gan yan*)

Chinese Herbs (Prescription)

Gentiana scabra, Scutellaria baicalensis, Gardenia jasminoides, Alisma plantago-aquatica, Akebia trifoliata, Plantago asiatica, Angelica sinensis, Bupleurum chinense, Glycyrrhiza uralensis, Rhemannia glutinosa (prescription: *long dan xie gan tang*).

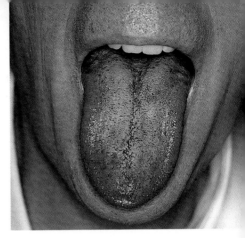

Fig. **123**: ▷ Character and color of the coating

Dietetic Treatment

- **To be avoided**

Avoid all kinds of alcohol in order to relieve the strain on the liver. Do not eat too sweet dishes because of their moistening properties.

- **Recommended diet**

Eat warm and neutral food from the earth element. Serve oysters that calm the liver and buckwheat from the warm fire element to detoxify the system.

The Thin, White Coating

Fig. **124**: The same patient as depicted in Figure **123** three weeks after starting treatment with acupuncture and herbal prescription. The Chinese differentiating syndrome diagnosis still is "wetness–heat within liver and gallbladder." However, this photograph shows that the white coating has become much thinner, which signifies a reduced accumulation of wetness in his system. The dark red color of the body of the tongue reveals that the very strong heat influence inside his organism still continues.

Therapy According to Syndrome Differentiation

> Nourish *yin*, cool heat, direct off liver–fire, and calm the mind (*shen*)

Chen Chiu Foramina

- SP-6
- LR-2 (3), LR-14
- BL-15, BL-18, BL-23, BL-25
- LI-11
- CV (*ren mai*)-4, CV-6, CV-14
- GV (*du mai*)-14

Chinese Herbs (Prescription)

Bupleurum chinense, Ostrea gigas, Anemarrhena asphodeloides, Paeonia lactiflora, Uncaria rhynchophylla, Ophiopogon japonicus, Scutellaria baicalensis, Glycyrrhiza uralensis.

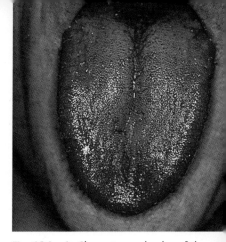

Fig. **124**:   ▷ Character and color of the coating

Dietetic Treatment

- **To be avoided**

Avoid hot food from the fire element, very hot spices, and too salty dishes. Avoid desiccating drinks such as coffee, red wine, alcohol, and spirits.

- **Recommended diet**

Serve oysters to calm the liver. Eat food from the wood element that nourishes the liver and from the water element that nourishes the kidney *yin*, for example seafood.

The Missing Coating with Red Tongue Body

Fig. **125**: This tongue reveals a marked emptiness of the stomach *qi* associated with a deficiency of the blood and *yin* in the interior. If the coating is completely missing, this indicates a severe disease. The reappearance of the coating on such a tongue indicates that the illness is receding.

Therapy According to Syndrome Differentiation

Strengthen *yin* and blood

Chen Chiu Foramina

- SP-6, SP-10
- CV (*ren mai*)-4, CV-6, CV-12
- BL-20, BL-23
- ST-36
- LI-11

Chinese Herbs (Prescription)

Rhemannia glutinosa, Astragalus membranaceus, Ophiopogon japonicus, Angelica sinensis, Glycyrrhiza uralensis.

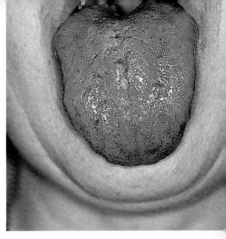

Fig. **125**: ▷ Character of the coating and color of the tongue body

Dietetic Treatment

- **To be avoided**

Avoid hot food from the fire elements as well as too hot and strong spices and too salty dishes. No drinks with a desiccating effect like coffee, red wine, brandy.

- **Recommended diet**

Eat vegetable soup with *Angelica sinensis* (one liter of water plus two spoons of Angelica root, to be cooked for 30 minutes).

The Red and Dry Tongue

Fig. **126**: This tongue documents the effect of a careless application of steroids over many years. It reveals the resulting severe exhaustion of the *yin*, which cannot even be treated successfully with Chinese medicine. Nevertheless, the condition of the patient had improved after acupuncture and herbal prescriptions, and her chronic bronchial asthma with wheezing subsided and cough attacks disappeared.

Therapy According to Syndrome Differentiation

Nourish *yin* and strengthen blood, open up the lung

Chen Chiu Foramina

- SP-6
- KI-3
- LU-1, LU-7

- BL-13, BL-15, BL-20, BL-23
- LI-11
- ST-36

Chinese Herbs (Prescription)

Angelica sinensis, Rhemannia glutinosa, Ephedra sinica, Atractylodes macrophala, Astragalus membranaceus, Pinellia ternata, Zingiber officinalis, Ophiopogon japonicus, Glycyrrhiza uralensis.

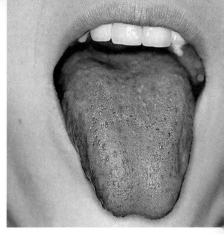

Fig. **126**: ▷ Color and consistency of the tongue body; character of the coating

Dietetic Treatment

- **To be avoided**

Avoid hot food from the fire element, for example grilled meat, brandy, bitter liqueurs, cognac.

- **Recommended diet**

Eat food from the metal element that strengthens the lungs, for example onions, mustard, cress, and food from the water element that reinforces the kidney such as seafood, algae (seaweed).

The Amorphous (Shapeless) Tongue

Fig. **127**: This tongue is without a structured consistency. It reveals a rugged and sticky coating, which is irregular and patchy. The body of the tongue is pale and slightly purple. The clinical diagnosis is lupus erythematosus. The 34-year-old patient suffered from extreme weakness of her body with generalized pain (fibromyalgia) after two twin pregnancies within only two years. Treatment by acupuncture was difficult because of her extreme exhaustion and led to an improvement only after six months of continued sessions once a week.

Therapy According to Syndrome Differentiation

Nourish and strengthen the essence (*jing*), strengthen spleen and kidneys, and dissolve phlegm (mucus)

Chen Chiu Foramina

- BL-20, BL-23
- ST-36
- SP-6, SP-9
- CV (*ren mai*)-4 (moxibustion!), CV-6, CV-12
- LI-4, LI-11
- HT-7

Chinese Herbs (Prescription)

Codonopsis pilulosa, Panax Ginseng, Atractylodes macrocephala, Rhemannia glutinosa, Dioscorea batatas, Pinellia ternata, Prunus persica, Angelica sinensis, Glycyrrhiza uralensis.

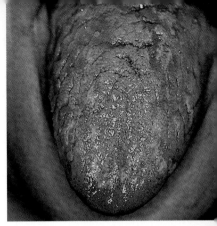

Fig. **127**: ▷ Color, character, and consistency of the tongue body;
character and consistency
of the coating

Dietetic Treatment

● **To be avoided**
Avoid food that causes the production of phlegm, particularly very
sweet food from the earth element, and too salty food leading to
the descent of humidity. Too sour food from the wood element
should equally be omitted because of its astringent properties.

● **Recommended diet**
Eat food from the metal element that opens up the surface and
dishes from the earth element that strengthen the spleen. Serve
compote made of Chinese red dates (*da zao, Fructus jujuba*, cf. Materia Medica, Group 19a, p. 291) with ginger and honey.

Pathological Appearance of the Tongue (1)

Fig. **128**: A markedly disturbed condition of the tongue with a thick, sticky, and yellow coating on the root, stamped out and missing coating on the left edge and at the tip ("map tongue"). The body of the tongue is fiery red. This patient suffers from shingles (herpes zoster) with severe intercostal neuralgia, insomnia, general nervousness, and irritation. Internal fire associated with an accumulation of phlegm (mucus) is the origin of this situation according to Chinese medicine.

Therapy According to Syndrome Differentiation

Dissolve phlegm (mucus) and extinguish internal fire

Chen Chiu Foramina

- ST-36, ST-40
- LI-4, LI-11
- BL-13, BL-15, BL-20, BL-23
- HT-7
- LR-2 (3), LR-14
- SP-6
- LU-1

Chinese Herbs (Prescription)

Pinellia ternata, Trichosanthes kirilowii, Ostrea gigas, Paeonia lactiflora, Stegodon orientalis, Uncaria rhynchophylla, Alisma plantago-aquatica, Poria cocos, Glycyrrhiza uralensis.

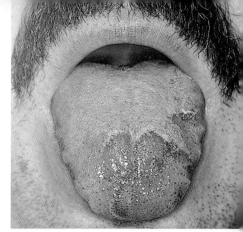

Fig. **128**: ▷ Color and shape of the
tongue body; color, char-
acter, and consistency of
the coating

Dietetic Treatment

- **To be avoided**

Avoid hot and desiccating food from the fire element, for example grilled meat and pungent spices. No cooking methods that reinforce *yang*.

- **Recommended diet**

Eat refreshing and cooling food from the wood element, for example products made of soured milk and tomatoes that reinforce
the liver. Serve oysters that calm the liver. Use cooking methods
that support *yin*. Use refreshing food from all elements. Recommended drinks: fresh water, Chinese green tea.

Pathological Appearance of the Tongue (2)

Fig. **129**: A red tip with generalized accumulation of phlegm within the middle and the lower burners. This condition is a heart–fire associated with weakness of spleen and stomach. The young woman suffers from insomnia, lack of appetite, and difficulty concentrating.

Therapy According to Syndrome Differentiation

Calm the heart and the mind (*shen*), dissolve phlegm, and strengthen the spleen

Chen Chiu Foramina

- BL-14, BL-15, BL-20, BL-23
- ST-36, ST-40
- SP-2, SP-6
- HT-3, HT-7
- GV (*du mai*)-14

Chinese Herbs (Prescription)

Pinellia ternata, Poria cocos, Trichosanthes kirilowii, Cinnamomum cassia, Ziziphus jujuba, Paeonia lactiflora, Glycyrrhiza uralensis.

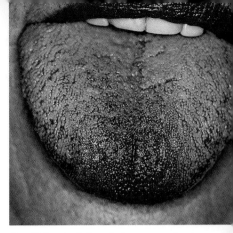

Fig. 129: ▷ Color of the tongue body; color, character, and consistency of the coating

Dietetic Treatment

- **To be avoided**

Avoid hot and desiccating food from the fire element, for example grilled meat and very spicy dishes. Do not use cooking methods that reinforce *yang*. No alcoholic beverages.

- **Recommended diet**

Eat food from the earth element that strengthens the spleen (potatoes, pumpkin, carrots). Serve food from the metal element which does not irritate the digestive tract and opens up the surface. Bitter-tasting food from the fire element can be served, in addition.

Pathological Appearance of the Tongue (3)

Fig. **130**: A slightly swollen tongue with a tip reddened by numerous protruding filiform papillae. The conventional diagnosis is insomnia, lack of concentration, and nervousness.

Therapy According to Syndrome Differentiation

Nourish *yin*, extinguish heart–fire, and strengthen spleen *yang*

Chen Chiu Foramina

- ST-36
- SP-6
- BL-20, BL-21
- HT-3
- LI-11
- GB-20

Chinese Herbs (Prescription)

Bupleurum chinense, Glycyrrhiza uralensis, Paeonia lactiflora, Poria cocos, Atractylodes macrocephala.

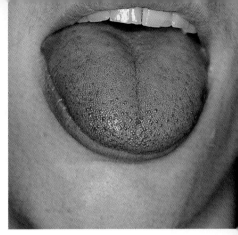

Fig. **130**: ▷ Color and shape of the
tongue body; consistency

Dietetic Treatment

- **To be avoided**

Avoid hot and desiccating food, for example strong alcoholic
drinks and grilled meat. Avoid very spicy dishes. Do not use cooking methods that reinforce *yang*.

- **Recommended diet**

Eat warm and hot food from the earth element that strengthen
the spleen *yang*. Use asparagus that nourishes *yin* and serve refreshing food from the fire element (e. g., chicory) in order to extinguish the fire of the heart. Apply cooking methods that reinforce the *yin*. Recommended beverages: Chinese green tea, fresh
water.

Pathological Appearance of the Tongue (4)

Fig. **131**: A large and red body of the tongue with a thin white coating. The center of this tongue is fissured (middle burner). The 55-year-old male patient complains of chronic indigestion, low back pain, and headache with irritability. His pulse is tense and floating. According to Chinese medicine this corresponds to a moderate blockage and accumulation of phlegm (mucus) in the organism.

Therapy According to Syndrome Differentiation

Strengthen the spleen, calm the liver, and dissolve phlegm (mucus)

Chen Chiu Foramina

- ST-36, ST-40
- SP-6
- BL-20, BL-21
- LI-11
- GB-20
- LR-3

Chinese Herbs (Prescription)

Bupleurum chinense, Pinellia ternata, Glycyrrhiza uralensis, Poria cocos, Atractylodes macrocephala, Paeonia lactiflora.

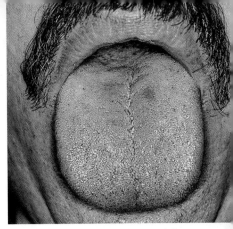

Fig. **131:** ▷ Color and shape of the
tongue body; character and
consistency of the coating

Dietetic Treatment

● **To be avoided**
Avoid hot and desiccating food from the fire element, especially
spicy dishes, grilled meat, and alcoholic drinks. Do not use cooking methods that reinforce *yang*.

● **Recommended diet**
Eat refreshing and cooling food from the wood element to calm
the liver. Serve oysters. Serve not too sweet food from the earth
element which strengthens the spleen, for example potatoes,
pumpkin, and carrots. Use food from the metal element that does
not irritate the digestive tract and opens up the surface.

Pathological Appearance of the Tongue (5)

Fig. **132**: Congested sublingual veins in a case of blood blockage (*yu xue*). This patient suffers from hypertension, stenocardia, varicose veins, and hemorrhoids following chronic low back pain. Chinese syndrome differentiation: Emptiness of the *yin* of kidneys and liver giving rise to liver *yang* and blockage of blood.

Therapy According to Syndrome Differentiation

> **Nourish kidney *yin*, lower liver *yang*, strengthen blood, and dissolve blood blockage**

Chen Chiu Foramina

- LI-4, LI-11
- BL-17, BL-18, BL-20, BL-23
- CV (*ren mai*)-4
- SP-6, SP-9, SP-10
- GV (*du mai*)-14
- LR-3, LR-14

Chinese Herbs (Prescription)

Carthamus tinctorius, Salvia miltiorrhiza, Curcuma longa, Curcuma zedoaria, Glechoma longituba, Prunus persica, Angelica sinensis, Glycyrrhiza uralensis, Dioscorea batatas, Rhemannia glutinosa.

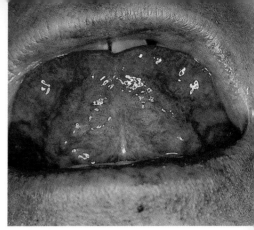

Fig. **132**

ietetic Treatment

To be avoided

void cooking methods that reinforce the *yang*. No food from the
re element, for example coffee.

Recommended diet

at food from the earth element. Use cooking methods that rein-
rce *yin*. Serve vegetable soup containing *Angelica sinensis* to
rengthen the blood.

6 Typical Topographic Changes of the Tongue in Relationship to Syndrome Differentiation (*Bian Zheng*)

In the following sections some typical changes of the tongue are documented and explained which are characteristic for certain pathological conditions involving the three burners (heaters) (cf. diagram inside the back cover).

- Tip of the tongue
- Margin of the tongue
- Area between tip and center
- Whole tongue
- Root of the tongue

The tip corresponds to the upper burner (heater), including heart and lungs.

Case 1 (Fig. **133**): Around age 45 years this patient developed emptiness of the heart *yin* and of the heart–blood (*xin xue xu*). Her complaints were palpitations, restlessness, insomnia, and sweating during the night. In conjunction with this, a round, shiny wart appeared on the end of her tongue. Her gynecologist had recommended treatment with estrogens, which had not brought about any improvement.

Therapy with acupuncture concentrated on nourishing the heart *yin* and the heart–blood. The patient was completely cured after 10 sessions. She is now without any symptoms, working full-time as a self-employed businesswoman, and needs no medication at all.

Therapy According to Syndrome Differentiation

> **Strengthen the heart *yin* and blood, and strengthen the kidney *yin***

Chen Chiu Foramina

- HT-3, HT-7
- PC-6
- SP-6, SP-10
- BL-15, BL-20, BL-23
- CV (*ren mai*)-6
- CV-12

Chinese Herbs (Prescription)

Scrophularia ningpoensis, Salvia miltiorrhiza, Poria cocos, Schizandra chinensis, Polygala tenuifolia, Platycodon grandiflorum, Angelica sinensis, Asparagus cochinchinensis, Ophiopogon japonicus, Biota orientalis, Ziziphus jujuba, Rhemannia glutinosa, Cinnabar, Panax Ginseng (prescription: *tian wang bu xin tang*).

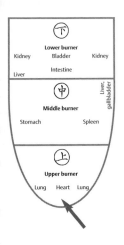

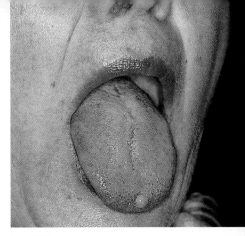

Fig. **133**

Dietetic Treatment

To be avoided

Avoid too salty dishes and hot food from the fire element like chillies, brandy, and grilled meat.

Recommended diet

Eat food that generates body liquids, especially from the earth and wood elements, for example wheat and morel cherries. Serve food which is not too salty from the water element to strengthen kidney *yin* (seafood, algae).

The margins of the tongue reflect the liver and gallbladder.

Case 2a (Fig. **134**): This female patient swallowed part of her false teeth, whereupon she was operated by emergency surgery at the university clinic in Göttingen. She received a blood transfusion contaminated with the hepatitis C virus. In the following, she developed a severe liver disease ending in liver cirrhosis. Her condition improved considerably during her treatment with acupuncture. Surgeons at the university clinic had told her that no therapy was available for her and that she would have to live with her disease.

Therapy According to Syndrome Differentiation

> **Dissolve blood blockage, nourish *yin* and blood, and activate the liver**

Chen Chiu Foramina

- LR-3, LR-14
- BL-17, BL-18, BL-23
- SP-6, SP-10
- CV (*ren mai*)-12, CV-14
- GV (*du mai*)-9, GV-14
- LI-11
- PC-6
- GB-20

Chinese Herbs (Prescription)

Carthamus tinctorius, Curcuma longa, Glechoma longituba, Salvia miltiorrhiza, Paeonia lactiflora, Angelica sinensis, and *Glycyrrhiza uralensis.*

Alternatively: *Gentiana scabra, Scutellaria baicalensis, Gardenia jasminoides, Alisma plantago-aquatica, Akebia trifoliata, Plantago asiatica, Angelica sinensis, Bupleurum chinense, Glycyrrhiza uralensis, Rhemannia glutinosa* (prescription: *long dan xie gan tang*).

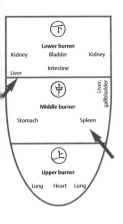

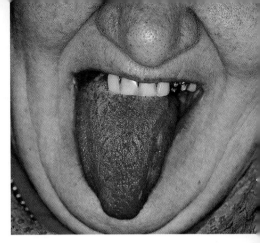

Fig. **134**

Dietetic Treatment

To be avoided

Avoid hot food from the fire element, for example coffee, all kinds of alcohol, as well as too greasy meals. Do not use cooking methods that reinforce *yang* (grilled meat, pickles, etc.).

Recommended diet

Eat food from the earth and wood elements that produce humidity. Taste: sweet and sour. Beverages: Drink a sufficient amount of water (two or three liters daily). Use cooking methods that reinforce *yin*.

Case 2b (Fig. **135**): According to Chinese tongue diagnosis the congested little bluish veins underneath the margin of the tongue signify a liver disease. For conventional Western medicine th
enlarged veins reveal a venous congestion in the pulmonary circu
lation brought about by the cirrhosis of the liver of this woma
(same case as on p. 207). At the onset of acupuncture treatment sh
complained of severe pain and pressure over her right hypochor
driac region, massive nycturia (nocturnal urination), and giddines
After five sessions all these symptoms had subsided.

Therapy According to Syndrome Differentiation

> **Dissolve blood blockage, nourish *yin*
> and blood, and activate the liver**

Chen Chiu Foramina

- LR-3, LR-14
- BL-17, BL-18, BL-23
- SP-6, SP-10
- CV (*ren mai*)-12, CV-14
- GV (*du mai*)-9, GV-14
- LI-11
- PC-6
- GB-20

Chinese Herbs (Prescription)

*Carthamus tinctorius, Curcuma longa, Glechoma longituba, Salvi
miltiorrhiza, Paeonia lactiflora, Angelica sinensis, Glycyrrhiza urale
sis.*
Alternatively: *Gentiana scabra, Scutellaria baicalensis, Gardeni
jasminoides, Alisma plantago-aquatica, Akebia trifoliata, Plantag
asiatica, Angelica sinensis, Bupleurum chinense, Glycyrrhiza urale
sis,* and *Rhemannia glutinosa* (prescription: *long dan xie gan tang*

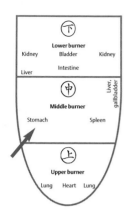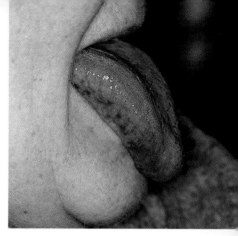

Fig. **135**

Dietetic Treatment

- **To be avoided**

Avoid hot food from the fire element, for example coffee, all kinds of alcohol, as well as too greasy meals. Do not use cooking methods that reinforce *yang* (grilled meat, pickles, etc.).

- **Recommended diet**

Eat food from the earth and wood elements that produce humidity. Taste: sweet and sour. Beverages: Drink a sufficient amount of water (two or three liters daily). Use cooking methods that reinforce *yin*.

Case 3 (Fig. **136**): This patient had suffered from bronchiectasis for many years with frequent attacks of bronchitis and chronic cough. The ulceration visible in the area of the upper burner reflects the inflammatory process in her lungs and bronchi. She received only little help from orthodox medicine. A series of acupuncture treatments changed her condition for the better. Her bronchial infections have since ceased; she is now able to work and lead a normal life.

Therapy According to Syndrome Differentiation

Strengthen the upper burner (lungs), dissolve phlegm (mucus), and strengthen the body's resistance (*wei qi*)

Chen Chiu Foramina

- LU-1, LU-5, LU-7
- ST-36, ST-40
- BL-12, BL-13, BL-20, BL-23
- CV (*ren mai*)-6

Chinese Herbs (Prescription)

Ephedra sinica, Atractylodes macrocephala, Paeonia lactiflora, Carthamus tinctorius, Zingiber officinale, Astragalus membranaceus, Pinellia ternata, Glycyrrhiza uralensis.

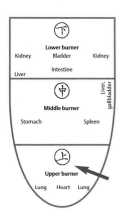
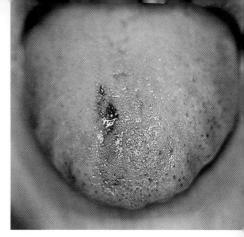

Fig. **136**

Dietetic Treatment

- **To be avoided**

Avoid desiccating food from the fire element (coffee, alcohol, red wine)

- **Recommended diet**

Eat food from the metal element that opens up the surface and dissolves phlegm, for example onions, horseradish, and mustard. Use herbs that warm up the internal organs and strengthen the body's resistance (*wei qi*), such as cinnamon, ginger, and fennel.

The color and consistency of the body of this tongue are both significant: Multiple fissures in conjunction with a dark red color of the whole tongue.

Case 4a (Fig. **137**): This young woman has a severe allergy against pollen (pollinosis), animal hair, and certain kinds of food. According to Chinese medicine she suffers from a *yin* deficiency with generalized internal fire (cf. Fig. **138**).

Therapy According to Syndrome Differentiation

Nourish *yin*, extinguish internal fire, and strengthen immunity (*wei qi*)

Chen Chiu Foramina

- LI-4, LI-11, LI-20
- BL-15, BL-20, BL-21, BL-23
- KI-3
- SP-6
- CV (*ren mai*)-4, CV-12

Chinese Herbs (Prescription)

Paeonia lactiflora, Poria cocos, Zingiber officinalis, Rhemannia glutinosa, Glycyrrhiza uralensis.

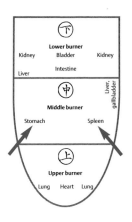

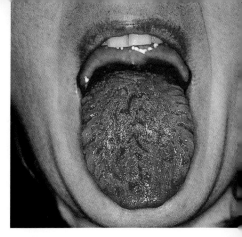

Fig. **137**

Dietetic Treatment

- **To be avoided**

Begin by excluding food intolerances or allergies. Avoid too spicy food, because this could trigger a heat condition (allergy). Preparation methods that reinforce cold, for example by freezing should be avoided, as well as food with too hot properties that stimulate internal fire in the organism.

- **Recommended diet**

Eat food with a warm character from all five elements, especially ginger, cinnamon, fennel (cf. Materia Medica, Group 10, p. 290). Use asparagus for reinforcing *yin*. Serve food from the earth element that strengthens the middle burner.

This disease is essentially constitutional, therefore the appearance of the tongue as shown in Figure 137 can only improve slowly.

Case 4b (Fig. **138**): After one initial treatment with acupuncture the allergic symptoms like rhinitis, conjunctivitis, nausea with vomiting after meals subsided. After four more sessions the patient was without complaints. The acupuncture treatment has, however, to be repeated annually because the entire system is involved.

Therapy According to Syndrome Differentiation

> Nourish *yin*, extinguish internal fire, and strengthen immunity (*wei qi*)

Chen Chiu Foramina

- LI-4, LI-11, LI-20
- BL-15, BL-20, BL-21, BL-23
- KI-3
- SP-6
- CV (*ren mai*)-4, CV-12

Chinese Herbs (Prescription)

Paeonia lactiflora, Poria cocos, Zingiber officinalis, Rhemannia glutinosa, Glycyrrhiza uralensis.

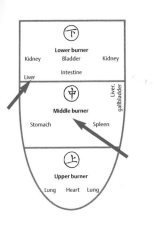

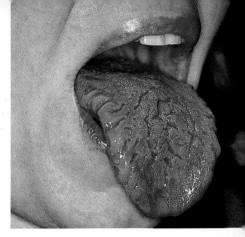

Fig. **138**

Dietetic Treatment

- **To be avoided**

Begin by excluding food intolerances or allergies. Avoid too spicy food, because this could trigger a heat condition (allergy). Preparation methods that reinforce cold, for example by freezing should be avoided, as well as food with too hot properties that stimulate the internal fire in the organism.

- **Recommended diet**

Eat food with a warm character from all five elements, especially ginger, cinnamon, fennel (cf. Materia Medica, Group 10, p. 290). Use asparagus for reinforcing *yin*. Serve food from the earth element to strengthen the middle burner.

The root of the tongue represents the lower burner (kidney, bladder, large intestine, genital organs).

Case 5 (Fig. **139**): A thick and sticky coating on the root of the tongue. The patient is an exhausted salesman with chronic lower back pain still persevering after two laminectomy operations. Eight treatments with acupuncture in conjunction with herbal prescription led to a marked improvement.

Therapy According to Syndrome Differentiation

Strengthen the kidney and the *qi*, and dissolve phlegm (mucus)

Chen Chiu Foramina

- BL-20, BL-23, BL-25
- ST-36, ST-40
- LI-4
- SP-9
- CV (*ren mai*)-4, CV-6
- GV (*du mai*)-3

Chinese Herbs (Prescription)

Rhemannia glutinosa, Alisma plantago-aquatica, Pinellia ternata, Poria cocos, Atractylodes macrocephala, Dioscorea batatas, Panax Ginseng, and *Glycyrrhiza uralensis.*

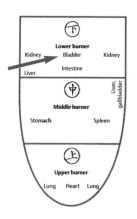

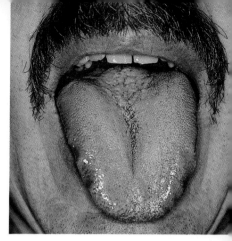

Fig. **139**

Dietetic Treatment

- **To be avoided**

Avoid cold dishes, uncooked and frozen food, ice-cream.

- **Recommended diet**

Eat warm meals from the earth and metal elements (leek, fennel, yellow paprika, pumpkin, and celery).

Case 6 (Fig. **140**): This young boy age 12 suffers from chronic tonsillitis and insomnia. His tongue reveals internal heat, especially in the upper burner (red and protruding filiform papillae on the tip) and in the lower burner (yellow coating), as well.

Therapy According to Syndrome Differentiation

> **Cool the heat and clean the lower burner**

Chen Chiu Foramina

- LU-1, LU-7, LU-11 (blood-letting)
- BL-12, BL-15, BL-23
- CV (*ren mai*)-6
- KI-3
- SP-6
- GV (*du mai*) -14
- SI-17

Chinese Herbs (Prescription)

Pueraria lobata, Ephedra sinica, Anemarrhena asphodeloides, Trichosanthes kirilowii, Paeonia lactiflora, Rhemannia glutinosa, Glycyrrhiza uralensis.

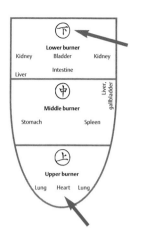

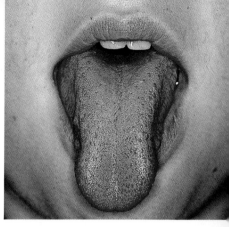

Fig. **140**

Dietetic Treatment

- **To be avoided**

Avoid hot and desiccating food, especially spirits, grilled meat, bitter and pungent spices.

- **Recommended diet**

Eat cold and refreshing food from the water element as it reinforces the kidney. Serve food from of the earth element. Use cooking methods that reinforce *yin*.

Multiple creases in the area corresponding to the middle burner.

Case 7 (Fig. **141**): This pale, delicate, and feeble tongue shows multiple creases in its center (middle burner). According to Chinese medicine the syndrome differentiation reveals an "emptiness of both heart and spleen" (*xin pi liang xu*).

Therapy According to Syndrome Differentiation

Strengthen the spleen and the heart

Chen Chiu Foramina

- ST-36
- SP-4
- CV (*ren mai*)-6, CV-12, CV-14
- BL-15, BL-20, BL-23
- HT-7

Chinese Herbs (Prescription)

Atractylodes macrocephala, Poria cocos, Astragalus membranaceus, Euphoria longan, Ziziphus spinosus (suan zao ren), Panax Ginseng, Saussura lappa, Glyzyrrhiza uralensis, Angelica sinensis, Polygala tenuifolia, Zingiber officinale, Ziziphus jujuba (da zao) (prescription: *gui pi tang*).

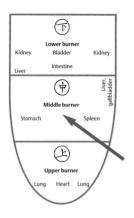
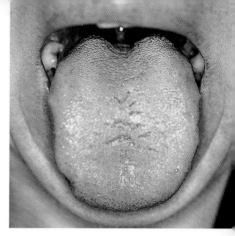

Fig. **141**

Dietetic Treatment

- **To be avoided**

Avoid hot food from the fire element as well as uncooked and frozen food.

- **Recommended diet**

Eat sweet-tasting food from the earth element as it strengthens spleen and stomach. Serve coarse wholemeal products. Use food from the fire element with neutral properties and a bitter taste to strengthen the heart, for example corn salad and brussels sprouts.

Case 8 (Fig. **142**): The whole tongue is covered with a thin, sticky coating, which corresponds to a generalized accumulation of liquid, as well as of cohesive phlegm (*tan yin*). The body of this tongue is pale, which indicates sensitivity to cold. This female patient suffers from bronchial asthma and mild mental depression associated with lower back pain.

Therapy According to Syndrome Differentiation

> **Dissolve phlegm (mucus), open up the bronchi, and strengthen spleen and kidney**

Chen Chiu Foramina

- LU-1, LU-7
- ST-36, ST-40
- PC-6
- BL-13, BL-23
- SP-6
- HT-7

Chinese Herbs (Prescription)

Pinellia ternata, Ephedra sinica, Panax Ginseng, Paeonia lactiflora, Zingiber officinalis, Rhemannia glutinosa, Glycyrrhiza uralensis, Astragalus membranaceus, and *Brassica alba.*

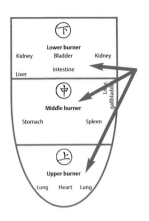

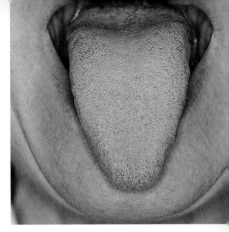

Fig. **142**

Dietetic Treatment

- **To be avoided**

Avoid cold food from all five elements. Do not use cooking methods that reinforce *yin*.

- **Recommended diet**

Eat warm food from the earth and water elements, for example chestnuts, pumpkin, potatoes, fish, and seafood.

Please note the thick coating on the root in conjunction with a red discoloration of the tip, rugged edges, and the daggerlike shape of this tongue.

Case 9 (Fig. **143**): This tongue is an example of a thick and sticky coating on the root associated with redness of the tip and an overall tenseness of the body. The 52-year-old woman suffers from marked mental depression with insomnia and deep-seated back pain. She has frequent bouts of cystopyelitis, in addition to spells of aggressive behavior.

Therapy According to Syndrome Differentiation

> Dissolve phlegm, calm heart and *shen*, calm the liver.

Chen Chiu Foramina

- ST-40
- BL-15, BL-18, BL-23, BL-25
- PC-6
- HT-7
- CV (*ren mai*)-4, CV-6
- LR-3

Chinese Herbs (Prescription)

Pinellia ternata, Bupleurum chinense, Uncaria rhynchophylla, Stegodon orientalis, Paeonia lactiflora, Poria cocos, Rhemannia glutinosa, Glycyrrhiza uralensis.

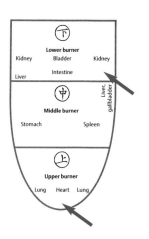
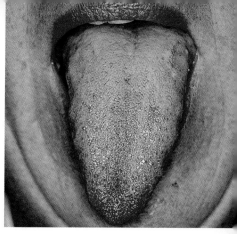

Fig. **143**

Dietetic Treatment

- **To be avoided**

Avoid hot and desiccating food, grilled meat, bitter and pungent spices, and, in particular, alcoholic drinks.

- **Recommended diet**

Eat cooling and refreshing food from the wood and fire elements, for example chicory and dandelion salad. Use cooking methods that reinforce *yin*. Serve asparagus that nourishes *yin*. Drink a sufficient amount of water in order to relieve the liver.

Case 10 (Fig. **144**): This tongue shows a fiery-red body with a sticky white coating in its center and on the root. The puffed up and bulging margins make the tongue look like a spoon. Conventional diagnoses: hypertension, liver disease following hepatitis, headache, dizziness.

Therapy According to Syndrome Differentiation

Calm the liver, excrete wind, dissolve phlegm (mucus), and expel heat

Chen Chiu Foramina

- LR-2 (3), LR-14
- LI-11
- BL-18, BL-23
- SP-6
- ST-36, ST-40
- GB-20
- GV (*du mai*)-14

Chinese Herbs (Prescription)

Bupleurum chinenese, Paeonia lactiflora, Ostrea gigas, Uncaria rhynchophylla, Trichosanthes kirilowii, Haliotis diversicolor, Atractylodes macrocephala, Glycyrrhiza uralensis.

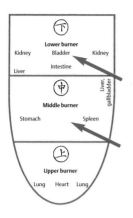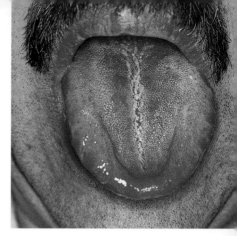

Fig. **144**

Dietetic Treatment

- **To be avoided**

Avoid hot food from the fire element, alcoholic drinks, and cooking methods that reinforce *yang* (grilling, roasting, barbecuing, pickling, etc.).

- **Recommended diet**

Eat food from the wood element, including oysters to calm the liver. Drink sufficient amounts of beverages made of soured milk, as well as fruit juices diluted with water (ratio 1:1) with a cooling effect.

7 Assessment of the Course of a Disease by Application of Tongue Diagnosis

The following figures document changes of the body, the coating, and the consistency of the tongue during the development of diseases, something which is of high clinical significance for adjusting therapeutic measures, as well as for prognosis.

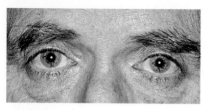

Fig. **145a**

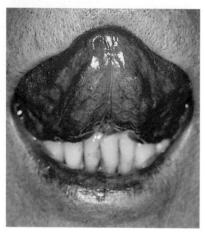

Fig. **145b**

Case 1: Life-Threatening NonA, NonB Hepatitis (Fig. 145a–i)

Fig. **145a, b**: This patient is the manager of a big German travel agency. He came with severe jaundice (the bilirubin was 23.7 mg/dL) after an infection with nonA, nonB hepatitis virus which he had contracted on a business trip while inspecting suitable hotels in South America. His infection did not respond to any conventional treatment and resulted in decompensated liver disease with initial liver cirrhosis. His consultant specialist, a university professor of gastroenterology, had suggested a liver transplant and told the patient that he would otherwise have to die within a few weeks. Apparently, he was petrified. That was 15 years ago (1988). Luckily, no donor for an organ transplant was available at that time and his physician referred him to an acupuncture specialist. That is why he is still alive today.

Fig. **145c–f**: After three sessions of acupuncture treatment the very high transaminases (around 600–800) normalized dramatically and the bilirubin came down to almost normal values. The patient's tongue and his eyes reflect the development in the various phases of the disease: The coating changed and disappeared. The extremely yellow inferior side of the tongue returned to a normal color. The influence of internal heat, reflected by the red color of the body, decreased. After three months of treatment by acupuncture and herbal therapy the patient was able to take up his responsible and demanding job.

For further development and summary of treatment see page 232 f.

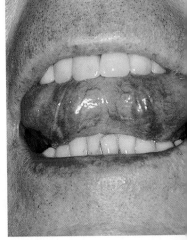

Fig. **145d**

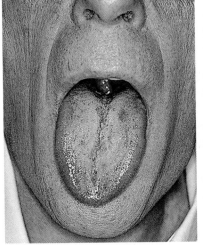

Fig. **145c**

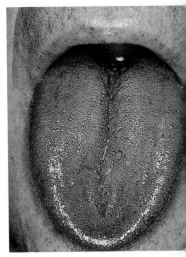

Fig. **145e**

Fig. **145f**

Fig. **145g, h**: One year after the onset of his disease he suffered from a relapse with extreme exhaustion, indigestion, associated with elevated bilirubin and transaminases in laboratory tests. Treatment with acupuncture and herbal prescriptions again brought him immediate remission of his symptoms. Four years after the outbreak of his severe infection he got married. Today he is enjoying good health, including normal laboratory values.

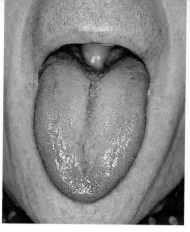

Fig. **145g**

Fig. **145i**: Normalized appearance of his tongue with a remaining red-

Therapy According to Syndrome Differentiation

Dissolve blood blockage, improve liver function (*shu gan*), cool internal heat, and excrete poison

Chen Chiu Foramina

- ST-36
- GB-34
- SP-6, SP-9

- LR-2, LR-3, LR-14
- BL-18, BL-19, BL-20, BL-23
- (alternating with BL-14, BL-15, BL-25)

- GV (*du mai*) -14, GV-20
- NP-88 (*gan yan*)

Chinese Herbs (Prescription)

Gentiana scabra, Scutellaria baicalensis, Gardenia jasminoides, Alisma plantago-aquatica, Akebia trifoliata, Plantago asiatica, Angelica sinensis, Bupleurum chinense, Glycyrrhiza uralensis, Rhemannia glutinosa (prescription: *long dan xie gan tang*).

Clinical Part

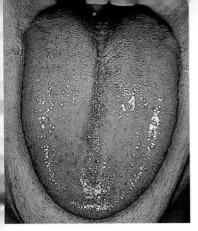

Fig. **145h**

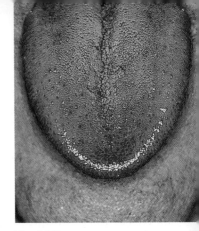

Fig. **145i**

dened (influence of internal heat) body of his tongue. This was six years after the photographs in Figures **144b** and **144e** were taken.

Alternating with: *Bupleurum chinense, Rhemannia glutinosa, Paeonia lactiflora, Ostrea gigas, Uncaria rhynchophylla, Prunus persica, Artemisia capillaris, Angelica sinensis, Glycyrrhiza uralensis, Atractylodes macrocephala, Codonopsis pilulosa, Trichosanthes kirilowii.*

Dietetic Treatment

- **To be avoided**

Avoid hot food and drinks from the fire element, specially alcohol and coffee.

- **Recommended diet**

Eat food from the wood element, for example tomatoes with balsamico, parsley, products made from soured milk such as cottage cheese. Serve oysters to calm the liver. Use food from the earth element that reinforces the middle burner.

Case 2: Chronic Lower Back Pain Resistant to Treatment (Fig. 146a, b)

This female patient for years suffered from severe back pain that was resistant to treatment by orthodox medicine. She came because of a relapse after an initially successful therapy with acupuncture three years previously. The body of her tongue is markedly red; the coating shows a black discoloration on the root in the area related to the lower burner, corresponding to the kidney and the lumbar spine. It must be remembered that in Chinese medicine all lower back pain conditions are related to kidney disorder. After five acupuncture treatments the black color of the coating had changed into a white-yellowish one. Simultaneously, she experienced marked relief of her back pain. The modification of her tongue indicates that a further improvement is to be expected.

Therapy According to Syndrome Differentiation

Nourish kidney *yin*, dissolve phlegm (mucus), and excrete internal heat

Chen Chiu Foramina

- BL-23, BL-25, BL-40, BL-52
- GV (*du mai*)-3, GV-9
- CV (*ren mai*)-6
- LI-4, LI-11

Chinese Herbs (Prescription)

Rhemannia glutinosa, Alisma plantago-aquatica, Angelica sinensis, Cornus officinalis, Dioscorea batatas, Rhemannia fermentata (shu di), Atractylodes macrocephala, Glycyrrhiza uralensis, Ziziphus jujuba, and *Pinellia ternata.*
Alternating with: *Rhemannia glutinosa, Poria cocos, Dioscorea batatas, Paeonia suffruticosa, Alisma plantago-aquatica, Cornus officinalis* (prescription: *liu wei di huang wan*).

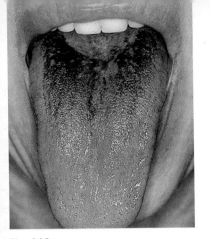

Fig. **146a**

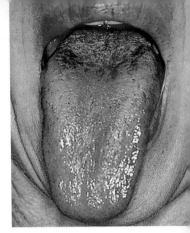

Fig. **146b**

Dietetic Treatment

● **To be avoided**

Avoid hot food from the fire element and cooking methods that reinforce *yang*. Drinks: No red wine, brandy, or coffee.

● **Recommended diet**

Eat food from the earth and water elements (seafood), and warm and neutral food from the metal element (garlic, ginger). Recommended drinks: sufficient amounts of water (two or three liters daily), Chinese green tea.

Case 3: Hypermenorrhea and Metromenorrhagie (Fig. 147a, b)

There is a time difference of approximately 25 years between the two photographs shown in Figures **147a** and **147b**. Initially, apart from an appendectomy, the young woman had been healthy except children's diseases such as measles, chicken pox, and mumps. Figure **147b** reveals the development of her health situation around age 45. Her tongue has become markedly red, which is typical for a *yin* deficiency, and it is considerably swollen. The red tongue indicates an emptiness of *yin* associated with rising emptiness–fire (*xu huo*). The swollen body with tooth marks at the same time signifies a *yang* deficiency. During the past 10 years she suffered from insomnia, constipation, and gynecological problems like hypermenorrhea and metromenorrhagia, a condition Chinese medicine refers to as heat–

Therapy According to Syndrome Differentiation

> **Nourish *yin* and blood extinguish internal heat, and reinforce *yang***

Chen Chiu Foramina

- SP-6, SP-10
- KI-3
- ST-36 (moxibustion)
- BL-15, BL-17, BL-23
- LI-4, LI-11
- HT-7
- CV (*ren mai*)-4
- GV (*du mai*)-14

Chinese Herbs (Prescription)

Ophiopogon japonicus, Asparagus cochinchinensis, Ziziphus jujuba, (red dates), *Angelica sinensis, Rhemannia glutinosa, Trichosanthes kirilowii,* and *Glycyrrhiza uralensis.*

fire in the lower burner, associated with myoma. Because of the myoma she was operated on twice, initially to remove the growth, and then, when the bleeding got out of control, a hysterectomy was carried out. She complains of mental depression, insomnia, nervousness, and night sweating. These are typical symptoms of an emptiness of *yin* associated with rising emptiness–fire which causes the red discoloration of her tongue. Her internal fire is quite strong and irritating, a condition motivating her to sleep with wide-open windows in the night, even in the cold wintertime. Consequently, she frequently suffers from cold attacks and flu.

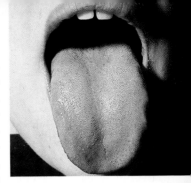

Fig. **147a**

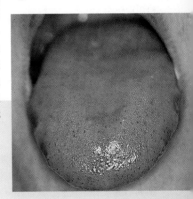

Fig. **147b**

Dietetic Treatment

- **To be avoided**

Avoid very hot and cold food and drinks, for example citrus fruits and bitter liqueur. Do not eat food from the fire element.

- **Recommended diet**

Eat cereals with a sweet taste (wheat, barley, buckwheat, millet), and soybean sprouts. Serve refreshing food from all five elements, in addition to uncooked food and milk products, with watermelon and cucumber.

Case 4: Hemiplegia after Cerebral Hemorrhage (Fig. 148a, b)

Fig. **148a, b**: The transition of a black coating into a yellow-brown-ish one, thus indicating an improvement of the hemiplegic condition. This patient suffers from the sequelae of a stroke (cerebral hemorrhage) resulting in a paralysis of his right side, both arm and leg. His hypoglossal nerve is not involved (cf. Changes of the Body, p. 273 f). For many years, he consumed one or two liters of red wine daily, a habit that got worse after he retired. Consequently, he gradually developed a strong and rising liver *yang* associated with weakening of his kidney *yin*, leading to the syndrome differentiation of liver–fire and, finally, to a liver–wind condition resulting in cerebral hemorrhage. He could only walk on crutches. The black coating of his tongue revealed an abundance of heat blocked in the interior of his organism, especially in the lower burner. After five acupuncture

Therapy According to Syndrome Differentiation

Nourish *yin*, calm and reinforce the liver, excrete heat and fire, expel wind

Chen Chiu Foramina

- ST-36, ST-37
- LI-4, LI-10, LI-11
- GB-20, GB-39
- BL-15, BL-18, BL-23
- LR-3, LR-14
- CV (*ren mai*)-6
- GV (*du mai*)-14, and GV-20

Chinese Herbs (Prescription)

Paeonia lactiflora, Uncaria rhynchophylla, Bupleurum chinense, Ostrea gigas, Haliotis diversicolor, Stegodon orientalis, Glycyrrhiza uralensis, Ophiopogon japonicus, Gypsum.

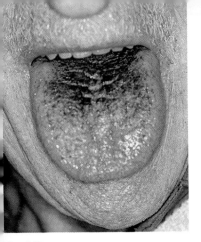
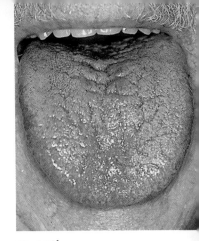

Fig. **148a**   Fig. **148b**

treatments the black coating was converted into a yellow-brownish one. Simultaneously, the overall condition of the patient had changed much to the better. He can now move both his arms and legs freely and is able to walk without a stick.

Alternating with: *Gastrodia elata, Uncaria rhynchophylla, Haliotis diversicolor, Gardenia jasminoides, Scutellaria baicalensis, Eucommia ulmoides, Leonurus heterophyllus, Loranthus parasiticus, Polygonum multiflorum, Poria cocos, Cyathula capitata (prescription: tian ma gou teng yin).*

Dietetic Treatment

- **To be avoided**

Avoid hot food from the fire element. Do not use cooking methods that reinforce *yang* (grilling, pickling). Drinks: No alcohol and coffee.

- **Recommended diet**

Eat oysters that calm the liver and asparagus that nourishes *yin*. Serve warm and refreshing food from the metal element. Use cooking methods that reinforce *yin*. Recommended drinks: Chinese green tea, fruit juices mixed with water.

8 Tongue Differentiation in Headache Patients

A Clinical Study of 14 Cases

In the following, 14 basically different tongue conditions are presented of patients with the orthodox Western diagnoses of headache, migraine, hemicrania, tension headache, cluster headache, etc. who came to our clinic from 1979 to 1999. They had without exception remained resistant to conventional therapy performed with painkillers, beta-blockers, and tranquilizers, as well as to insufficient acupuncture procedures applied according to Western diagnoses without diagnostic evaluation of the individual syndrome. Figures **149–162** clearly show *why* these inadequate therapies had remained without favorable results: Only the abstract term "headache" had been aimed at in the foreground without regarding the real condition of the individual patient as a whole living being. Thus, the insufficient treatment did not meet the requirements of a truly scientific procedure (cf. Summary and Outlook, p. 278).

All 14 patients were cured of their headache or migraine in our clinic despite the poor results they had experienced before. It should be mentioned that our acupuncture and herbal treatment was geared to individual syndrome differentiation and that mainly foramina on the body, the arms, and legs were used, and only very few sites on the head were acupunctured. In other words: The real cause of most cases of headache or migraine is not to be found on or in the head and its structures, but inside the organism and the internal organs.

The time required for a successful completion of acupuncture and herbal therapy amounted on average to two to three months with 10 to 15 individual treatment sessions.

Case 1 (Fig. 149)

This is a light white and slightly swollen tongue with multiple little creases in the middle, which refers to the middle burner representing spleen and stomach. The patient is very susceptible to cold. The character of his headache is deep and dull; the pain worsens in cold weather.

According to Chinese medicine this is a case of emptiness of the spleen *yang*.

Therapy According to Syndrome Differentiation

Strengthen the spleen, warm up the *yang*, and dissolve wetness (damp)

Chen Chiu Foramina

- ST-25 (moxibustion), ST-36
- SP-6, SP-9
- CV (*ren mai*)-4, CV-6, CV-12
- LI-11

Chinese Herbs (Prescription)

Atractylodes macrocephala, Zingiber officinalis, Dioscorea batatas, Eucommia ulmoides, Poria cocos, Cinnamomum cassia, and *Glycyrrhiza uralensis.*

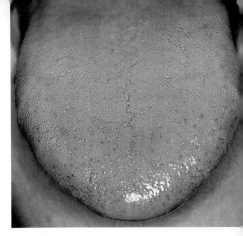

Fig. **149**

Dietetic Treatment

- **To be avoided**

Avoid cold food with a cold character and cooking methods that reinforce *yin*, ice-cream, and tropical fruits. Avoid all kinds of sprouts, fruit juice, button mushrooms, algae (seaweed).

- **Recommended diet**

Eat warm food from the earth element, for example rice, fennel, chestnut, pumpkin. Use walnuts to reinforce *yang* (cf. Chinese Materia Medica, Group 19b, p. 291)

Case 2 (Fig. 150)

This is a reddened tongue with thin white coating and a slightly reddened tip. The edges on both sides of the body are swollen and red the coating is partly missing on their upper right side. The headache is related to this young female patient's monthly menstrual bleeding; its character is burning and stabbing. The patient suffers, in addition, from insomnia.

The syndrome differentiation is *yin* emptiness with rising liver *yang*, and heart–fire.

Therapy According to Syndrome Differentiation

> **Nourish *yin*, strengthen blood, and calm liver (*ping gan*) and heart (*an xin*)**

Chen Chiu Foramina

- SP-6, SP-10
- LR-3
- KI-3
- BL-15, BL-18, BL-23
- HT-3, HT-7
- CV (*ren mai*)-4, CV-14
- GV (*du mai*)-14

Chinese Herbs (Prescription)

Angelica sinensis, Ophiopogon japonicus, Bupleurumn chinense, Paeonia lactiflora, Ziziphus jujuba, Poria cocos, Equus asinus, and *Glycyrrhiza uralensis.*

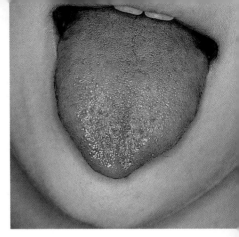

Fig. **150**

Dietetic Treatment

- **To be avoided**
Avoid hot food from the metal and fire elements, and cooking methods that reinforce *yang*. Do not use too hot (metal) and too bitter (fire) food.

- **Recommended diet**
Eat oysters to calm the liver (Chinese Materia Medica, Group 11, p. 290); use two spoons of *Angelica sinensis* root per one liter of chicken or vegetable broth, cook for 30 minutes. Serve asparagus and refreshing food from the wood element, in addition to neutral food from the fire element like corn salad, brussels sprouts, or arugula salad.

Case 3 (Fig. 151)

This tongue is covered all over with a sticky white coating which is caused by a spleen weakness and emptiness with accumulation of wetness and phlegm. Consequently, the clear *yang* cannot rise upward to the head. Such a condition results in bouts of oppressing pain sensation on the level of the head, associated with a sensation of fullness in the epigastric region, and heavy arms and legs.

Chinese medicine refers to this condition as a headache caused by a blockage of phlegm and wetness.

Therapy According to Syndrome Differentiation

> **Strengthen the spleen, dissolve and excrete phlegm and wetness**

Chen Chiu Foramina

- SP-6, SP-9
- ST-21, ST-40
- CV (*ren mai*)-4, CV-12
- BL-15, BL-20, BL-21
- GV (*du mai*)-20

Chinese Herbs (Prescription)

Pinellia ternata, Atractylodes macrocephala, Astragalus membranaceus, Poria cocos, Grifola umbellata, and *Glycyrrhiza uralensis.*

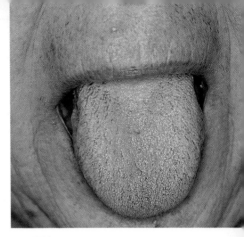

Fig. **151**

Dietetic Treatment

- **To be avoided**

Avoid cold food from the wood element, for example tomato. Do not use cooking methods that reinforce *yin*; no ice-cream.

- **Recommended diet**

Eat food from the metal element and neutral and warm food from the earth element like cereals, pumpkin, carrots.

Case 4 (Fig. 152)

This tongue is very red; its margin is puffed up and reveals a network of thin veins especially on the inferior side of the body. The patient, an overworked and exhausted salesman, complains of a headache moving from his forehead to the vertex and from here to the back of his neck. He suffers from attacks of dizziness associated with scintillating scotoma.

Chinese medicine refers to this condition as liver *yang* syndrome with the tendency to transform into liver–fire. In the background this disturbance is triggered by a weakened *yin* producing internal fire associated with wind. Both fire and wind are *yang* disorders and as such have the tendency to rise upward and to accumulate on the level of the head. This causes intracranial blood congestion. In addi-

Therapy According to Syndrome Differentiation

Calm the liver, extinguish pathological fire and wind, and stimulate blood circulation within the liver

Chen Chiu Foramina

- LR-3, LR-14
- BL-18, BL-23
- ST-36
- GV (*du mai*)-14, GV-20
- GB-8, GB-20
- LI-4, LI-11
- SP-10

Chinese Herbs (Prescription)

Bupleurum chinense, Paeonia lactiflora, Ostrea gigas, Angelica sinensis, Curcuma zedoaria, Uncaria rhynchophylla, Ophiopogon japonicus, Trichosanthes kirilowii, and *Glycyrrhiza uralensis.*

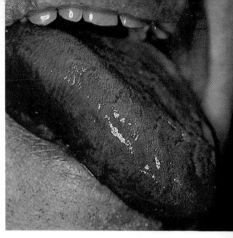

Fig. **152**

tion, there is an accumulation of blood in the liver. Climatic influences of windy weather with an approaching storm or gale usually give rise to a worsening of his headache. Therefore, the man is extremely susceptible to wind and tries to avoid draughty environments. In between his attacks the pain concentrates on one spot of his right temple, which motivated conventional neurologists to diagnose a "cluster headache." Another orthodox diagnosis of his disease was "fatty infiltration of the liver," for which condition was no specific treatment available.

Dietetic Treatment

- **To be avoided**

Avoid hot food from the metal and fire elements. Refrain from drinking all sorts of alcohol. Do not eat crabmeat because of its adverse effect in cases of wind disease.

- **Recommended diet**

Eat neutral food from the wood element such as leek, celery, fresh juice prepared with celery. Recommended drink: sufficient fresh water.

Case 5 (Fig. 153)

This tongue is completely covered with a sticky, white coating, which is especially thick on the root, thus representing phlegm within the lower burner. The female patient suffers from drowsiness associated with oppressing pain in her head. In addition, she complains of heavy limbs and chronic lumbago with severe lower back pain.

Chinese medicine analyses this clinical condition as an accumulation of wetness–phlegm within the lower and middle burners.

Therapy According to Syndrome Differentiation

> **Dissolve and excrete phlegm and wetness, strengthen the spleen, and warm kidney *yang***

Chen Chiu Foramina

- ST-36, ST-40
- SP-6, SP-9
- CV (*ren mai*)-6, CV-9
- BL-20, BL-23 (moxibustion!), BL-40
- GV (*du mai*)-3

Chinese Herbs (Prescription)

Pinellia ternata, Poria cocos, Atractylodes macrocephala, Glycyrrhiza uralensis.
Alternating with: *Aconitum carmichaeli, Poria cocos, Grifola umbellata, Paeonia lactiflora, Atractylodes macrocephala, Zingiber officinale* (prescription: *zhen wu tang*).

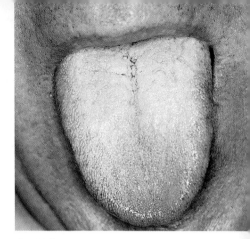

Fig. **153**

Dietetic Treatment

- **To be avoided**

Avoid astringent food from the wood element that contracts humidity in the system, for example pickled gherkins, sauerkraut. No cold food from the water element, for example algae (seaweed).

- **Recommended diet**

Eat neutral and warm food from the earth element and leeks fried with walnuts to reinforce kidney *yang*.

Case 6 (Fig. 154)

This red tongue with swollen edges shows a slightly protruding and intensely red tip and a yellow coating in its central crease. Filiform papillae have turned into fungiform and reddened ones, indicating strong internal heat.

This patient's headache travels from both eyes to his nape. He is very irritable with frequent outbreaks of rage and he suffers from insomnia. This is a very strong liver–fire associated with heart–fire in addition to an accumulation of phlegm in the spleen and stomach.

Therapy According to Syndrome Differentiation

> **Calm the liver, excrete fire from liver and heart, expel wind, strengthen the spleen, and dissolve and excrete phlegm and wetness**

Chen Chiu Foramina

- LR-2 (3), LR-14
- ST-25, ST-40
- BL-15, BL-18, BL-20, BL-23
- LI-4, LI-11
- SP-6
- CV (*ren mai*)-12, CV-14
- GV (*du mai*)-14
- GB-20

Chinese Herbs (Prescription)

Angelica sinensis, Rheum palmatum, Coptis chinensis, Scutellaria baicalensis, Phellodenron amurense, Gentiana scabra, Aloe vera, Saussura lappa, Moschus moschiferus, Gardenia jasminoides Ellis, Isatis tinctoria, Zingiber officinale, Zizphus jujuba (prescription: *dang gui long hui wan*).

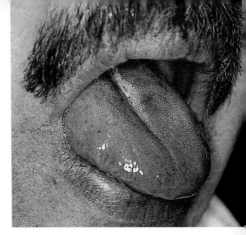

Fig. **154**

Dietetic Treatment

- **To be avoided**

Avoid hot food from all five elements, in particular food from the fire element, for example coffee, red wine, chillies.

- **Recommended diet**

Serve oysters to calm the liver. Eat cold and refreshing food from the wood element in addition to neutral food from the earth element to strengthen the spleen.

Case 7 (Fig. 155)

This tongue is red without a coating except a very thin layer close to the root. It has a narrowed and tense, bright red tip resembling a short bottleneck, which shows a cluster of protruding red papillae. The patient, an elderly woman, suffers from burning headache with insomnia in conjunction with a dry, titillating cough, and generalized weakness and tiredness.

According to Chinese medicine this is an emptiness of the *yin* of the heart and the kidneys associated with a mild emptiness of the *yin* of the lung. Such a syndrome differentiation is called "heart and kidney are not interconnected" (*xin shen bu jiao*).

Therapy According to Syndrome Differentiation

Strengthen kidney *yin* and heart *yin*, calm *shen*, and open up lung and bronchi

Chen Chiu Foramina

- KI-3
- SP-6
- BL-13, BL-15, BL-23
- CV (*ren mai*)-4, CV-6
- LU-1
- HT-3, HT-7
- ST-36

Chinese Herbs (Prescription)

Cinnamomum cassia, Ziziphus jujuba, Ophiopogon japonicus, Astragalus membranaceus, Rhemannia glutinosa, Ephedra sinica, Glycyrrhiza uralensis, and *Atractylodes macrocephala.*

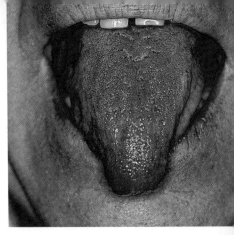

Fig. **155**

Alternating with: *Scrophularia ningpoensis, Salvia miltiorrhiza, Poria cocos, Schizandra chinensis, Polygala tenuifolia, Platycodon grandiflorum, Angelica sinensis, Asparagus cochinchinensis, Ophiopogon japonicus, Biota orientalis, Ziziphus jujuba, Rhemannia glutinosa, Cinnabar, Panax Ginseng* (prescription: *tian wang bu xin tang*).

Dietetic Treatment

- **To be avoided**

Avoid desiccating food from the fire element (coffee, red wine, very bitter food), as well as food with warm and hot properties.

- **Recommended diet**

Eat refreshing, slightly salty or bitter food and food from the earth element to produce humidity within the organism, for example wheat, millet, sesame, dairy products. Drink sufficient amounts of water (two or three liters daily). Use refreshing and neutral food from the metal element, for example red radish, horseradish, cabbage, turnip (kohlrabi).

Case 8 (Fig. 156)

This tongue has a red tip and is covered with a thin, white, and sticky coating involving all three burners. The patient suffers from a dull and agonizing headache with mental depression and diarrhea early in the morning around 5 o'clock. She is very susceptible to cold, suffers from paroxysmal palpitation and insomnia.

The analysis of this tongue in conjunction with other clinical signs reveals a blockage of phlegm associated with an emptiness of spleen *yang* and kidney *yang*. There is an additional emptiness of heart *qi* irritating the *shen*.

Therapy According to Syndrome Differentiation

> **Warm spleen *yang* and kidney *yang*, dissolve and excrete phlegm, and calm the heart *shen***

Chen Chiu Foramina

- ST-36, ST-40
- SP-4, SP-6
- CV (*ren mai*)-6, CV-12
- BL-15, BL-20, BL-23 (moxibustion!)
- HT-7

Chinese Herbs (Prescription)

Pinellia ternata, Trichosanthes kirilowii, Poria cocos, Grifola umbellata, Ziziphus jujuba (red dates), *Atractylodes macrocephala,* and *Glycyrrhiza uralensis.*
Alternating with: *Aconitum carmichaeli, Panax Ginseng, Zingiber officinale, Atractylodes macrocephala, Glycyrrhiza uralensis* (prescription: *fu zi li zhong wan*).

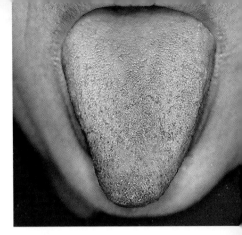

Fig. **156**

Dietetic Treatment

- **To be avoided**
Avoid food with cold properties. No coffee or black tea.

- **Recommended diet**
Eat warm food from the earth and water elements, for example fennel, pumpkin, leeks, onions. Use soybeans that eliminate humidity and dissolve phlegm.

Case 9 (Fig. 157)

This is a fiery red tongue. In fact, according to Chinese medicine, fire is the main element in its pathogenesis. A wide gap in the middle divides the tongue into two separate halves involving all the three burners. A thick, white, and sticky coating is spread over the root.

The patient's main complaint is a stabbing, fiery, and burning headache. He is extremely irritable with fits of anger and rage. He suffers from a dry mouth and is very thirsty. He frequently has a burning sensation in his eyes. He takes conventional medication because of hypertension.

Therapy According to Syndrome Differentiation

Calm the liver, nourish kidney *yin*, and extinguish liver–fire

Chen Chiu Foramina

- LR-2 (3)
- KI-3
- CV (*ren mai*)-6, CV-12
- LI-4, LI-6
- BL-15, BL-18, BL-23
- GB-20 (named *feng-chi*, "pool of the wind")
- GV (*du mai*)-14

Chinese Herbs (Prescription)

Paeonia lactiflora, Bupleurum chinense, Anemarrhena asphodeloides, Rhemannia glutinosa, Uncaria rhynchophylla, Ostrea gigas, Pinellia ternata, Glycyrrhiza uralensis.

Chinese medicine analyses this clinical condition as a strong liver–fire associated with kidney *yin* emptiness and an accumulation of phlegm in the middle and lower burners.

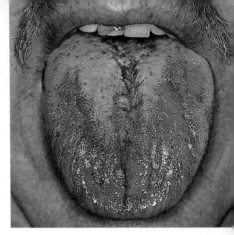

Fig. **157**

Alternating with: *Angelica sinensis, Rheum palmatum, Coptis chinensis, Scutellaria baicalensis, Phellodendron amurense, Gentiana scabra, Aloe vera, Saussura lappa, Moschus moschiferus, Gardenia jasminoides Ellis, Isatis tinctoria, Zingiber officinale, Ziziphus jujuba* (prescription: *dang gui long hui wan*).

Dietetic Treatment

- **To be avoided**
Avoid warm and hot food from the fire element, for example coffee, spirits, grilled meat.

- **Recommended diet**
Eat oysters to calm the liver (Chinese Materia Medica, Group 11b, p. 290) and refreshing food from the wood element. Recommended drinks: Sufficient amounts of water, Chinese green tea.

Case 10 (Fig. 158)

This tongue is covered with a thin, white coating and shows multiple transverse as well as some longitudinal creases in the area of the middle burner and red granular papillae on the tip. The patient's headache occurs mainly during the night and is associated with palpitations and spells of insomnia.

According to Chinese medicine this reveals an emptiness of the spleen *qi* with accumulation of wetness in the whole organism. The red tip signifies an ensuing emptiness of the heart with an onset of heart–fire.

Therapy According to Syndrome Differentiation

> **Strengthen the spleen, excrete wetness, and calm the heart**

Chen Chiu Foramina

- SP-6, SP-9
- ST-29, ST-36
- CV (*ren mai*)-6, CV-12, CV-14
- BL-15, BL-20, BL-21, BL-23
- HT-7
- LI-11

Chinese Herbs (Prescription)

Pinellia ternata, Poria cocos, Grifola umbellata, Atractylodes macrocephala, Stegodon orientalis, Angelica sinensis, Astragalus membranaceus, Zingiber officinale, Ziziphus spinosus, Glycyrrhiza uralensis.

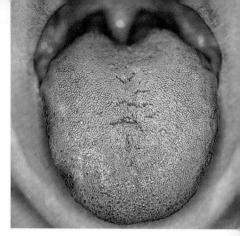

Fig. **158**

Dietetic Treatment

- **To be avoided**

Avoid hot food from the fire element, for example coffee. Do not use cooking methods that reinforce *yang*.

- **Recommended diet**

Eat compote of *Fructus jujuba* (Chinese red dates). Serve neutral food from the earth element. Serve neutral and refreshing food from the fire element, for example chicory, salad of radicchio and dandelion leaves. Drink chocolate (cocoa).

Case 11 (Fig. 159)

This is a thin, small tongue which is light in color, a condition indicating deficiency of both blood and *qi* (*xue qi*). Numerous creases in the center reveal that the spleen is in a condition of emptiness. A yellowish-gray and sticky coating covers the root. The patient, a university student, is very susceptible to cold. He suffers from severe bouts of headache, especially in wintertime and in cold surroundings. In addition, he complains of chronic pain in his knee joints, and he was diagnosed a chronic and relapsing prostatitis by a urologist who prescribed antibiotics. An orthopedic surgeon performed an arthroscopy of his knee joints and tried to "clean" the tendons and menisci, a procedure which did not produce a result. The young man suffers from attacks of anxiety and depression.

Therapy According to Syndrome Differentiation

Strengthen kidney *yang* (moxibustion!), strengthen the spleen, and excrete wetness from the lower burner

Chen Chiu Foramina

- BL-15, BL-20, BL-40
- BL-23, BL-51 (moxibustion!)
- ST-36, ST-40
- CV (*ren mai*)-3, CV-6
- KI-7
- SP-6
- GV (*du mai*)-1
- HT-7
- PC-6

Chinese Herbs (Prescription)

Atractylodes macrocephala, Panax Ginseng, Rhemannia glutinosa, Pinellia ternata, Alisma plantago-aquatica, Poria cocos, Cervus nippon, and *Glycyrrhiza uralensis.*

According to Chinese medicine this is a coldness syndrome associated with an emptiness of the kidney *yang* and accumulation of turbid wetness in the lower burner.

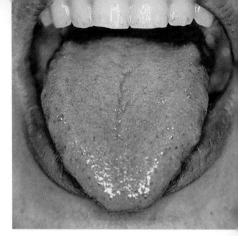

Fig. **159**

Dietetic Treatment

- **To be avoided**

Avoid cold food from all five elements. No coffee. Do not use cooking methods that reinforce *yin*. Avoid ice-cream and frozen food.

- **Recommended diet**

Eat walnuts that strengthen *yang* and leeks roasted with walnuts. Use fennel, white cabbage, and warm grape juice or blackcurrant juice.

Case 12 (Fig. 160)

This tongue is slightly swollen and shows multiple small fissures in its center and a thin powdery coating in the middle part and on the root. The tip is covered with red granular papillae. The old woman suffers from burning headaches associated with night sweating, back pain, palpitations, and insomnia.

By syndrome differentiation according to Chinese medicine an emptiness of *yin* with rising emptiness–fire can be diagnosed.

Therapy According to Syndrome Differentiation

Nourish *yin* and extinguish pathological fire

Chen Chiu Foramina

- SP-6
- KI-3
- GB-20
- BL-14, BL-15, BL-23, BL-40
- HT-3, HT-7
- ST-36
- CV (*ren mai*)-4

Chinese Herbs (Prescription)

Ophiopogon japonicus, Asparagus cochinchinensis, Angelica sinensis, Rheum palmatum, Gypsum, Glycyrrhiza uralensis.

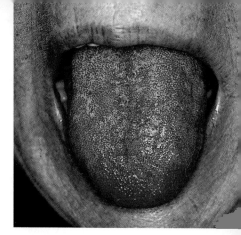

Fig. **160**

Dietetic Treatment

- **To be avoided**

Avoid hot and warm food from the fire and metal elements.

- **Recommended diet**

Use cooking methods that reinforce *yin*. Eat neutral and refreshing food from all five elements. Serve asparagus that nourishes *yin*. Ensure you get sufficient sleep to strengthen *yin*.

Case 13 (Fig. 161)

The color of this tongue is light. It reveals small tooth marks on the margin and a long and deep longitudinal gap in the middle. The root is covered with a gray, sticky coating.

The patient, a woman in her mid-forties, has suffered from severe migraine since her adolescence, which is associated with vomiting, stomach pain, and shivering fits before the outbreak of a headache attack. Further complaints are chronic back pain with ischialgia.

The differentiating syndrome diagnosis reveals a cold syndrome of the spleen and stomach, emptiness of kidney *yang*, and accumulation of phlegm and wetness in the middle and lower burners.

Therapy According to Syndrome Differentiation

Warm spleen *yang*, strengthen kidney *yang*, and excrete wetness and phlegm from the middle and lower burners

Chen Chiu Foramina

- SP-6, SP-9
- CV (*ren mai*)-6, CV-12 (moxibustion!)
- BL-20, BL-21, BL-23 (moxibustion!)
- PC-6
- KI-7

Chinese Herbs (Prescription)

Atractylodes macrocephala, Panax Ginseng, Angelica sinensis, Pinellia ternata, Bupleurum chinense, Dioscorea batatas, and *Glycyrrhiza uralensis.*

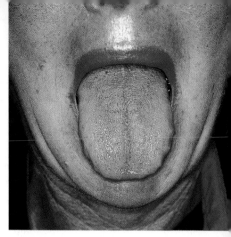

Fig. **161**

Dietetic Treatment

- **To be avoided**

Avoid cooking methods that reinforce *yin*. Avoid all kinds of cold
and refreshing food. No uncooked and frozen food; no ice-cream.

- **Recommended diet**

Use cooking methods and dishes that reinforce kidney *yang*, for
example roasted leek with walnuts. Eat warm food from the earth
element and warm cereals prepared from buckwheat. Eat soybeans and vegetables and spices with hot and warm properties
such as garlic, chillies, paprika, ginger, and coriander.

Case 14 (Fig. 162)

This young man's tongue shows signs of discrete tooth marks and a deep longitudinal crease in the center, in addition to a gray coating and a pink tip with protruding filiform papillae. The root is covered with numerous fiery red circumvallated papillae. The patient complains of a dull, tormenting headache, lack of appetite, nervousness, insomnia, back pain, and premature ejaculation during sexual intercourse.

The Chinese syndrome diagnosis reveals a joint emptiness of spleen and stomach, and of kidney and heart associated with wetness, heat and phlegm accumulated in the lower and middle burners.

Therapy According to Syndrome Differentiation

> **Strengthen spleen and stomach, dissolve phlegm, strengthen the kidney, excrete heat from the lower burner, and calm the heart and the *shen***

Chen Chiu Foramina

- ST-36
- BL-15, BL-20, BL-21, BL-23, BL-25
- CV (*ren mai*)-6, CV-12, CV-14
- SP-6, SP-9
- HT-7

Chinese Herbs (Prescription)

Paeonia lactiflora, Atractylodes macrocephala, Astragalus membranaceus, Ziziphus jujuba (red dates), *Panax Ginseng, Rhemannia glutinosa, Pinellia ternata, Zingiber officinalis,* and *Glycyrrhiza uralensis.*

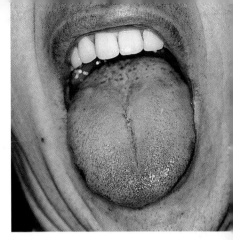

Fig. **162**

Dietetic Treatment

- **To be avoided**
Avoid food from the fire and metal elements.

- **Recommended diet**
Eat neutral and refreshing food from the earth element, in addition to vegetables and warm cereal dishes. Use roots of vegetable and pumpkin. Serve celery that reinforces the kidney.

9 Modern Research on Tongue Diagnosis

Over the last few decades, traditional Chinese tongue diagnostic has been scrutinized by the application of modern Western medical theories. Since the mid-seventies this research was, for example, carried out at the German Research Institute of Chinese Medicine (GRICMED), Freiburg im Breisgau/Germany. This research has produced the following results.

The Appearance of a Normal Tongue

Interpretation of a Normal Tongue

Under normal conditions, the tongue varies in color from pink to red since the tongue muscles and its mucous membranes are morphologically well supplied with blood vessels. Moreover, the tongue is covered in a thin and white coating as already pointed out in the above. This normal white layer consists of the tips of threadlike filiform papillae (papillae filiformes), often split at their end, and mushroom-shaped fungiform papillae (papillae fungiformes), in addition to food particles, saliva, and bacteria.

Changes in the Appearance of the Tongue

Changes of the Body

Any change in the color of the tongue body is closely related to the blood circulation within the organ. A whitish tongue indicates a reduction in the amount of blood, an anemia, or edematous swelling of the tongue body. In such cases the blood vessels shrink, the circulation slows down, and there is an insufficient blood supply in general. Chinese medicine relates this condition as emptiness of *yang*, of *qi*, or of blood.

In contrast to this, a dark red tongue signals that the blood vessels have enlarged in their capacity and that blood has accumulated in the tongue body. A bluish or purple discoloration of the tongue is related to a venous blood stagnation in the tongue or a general lack of oxygen in the organism. In such cases the sublingual veins appear thickened and darker than normal and the inferior side of the tongue should, therefore, be inspected during the examination. The purple color can be related to a lack of oxygen within the red blood cells contained in the blood vessels of the tongue. Orthodox medicine refers to this condition as cyanosis.

If a tongue is thick, soft, and swollen this can be due to a decrease in protein in the blood plasma. This causes a drop in the colloid osmotic pressure (water-attracting force of the blood). Thus, plasma fluids escape from the blood vessels into the tongue tissues, so forming an edema. This causes the enlargement of the tongue, which swells to the point of touching the teeth so that they leave marks on the edges of the tongue. An increase in the size of the tongue can also be caused by an abnormal relaxation of the tongue muscles. In addition, the lymphatic and venous drainage may be impaired, thus causing a swelling of the tongue body.

Fissures in the tongue occur when the filiform and fungiform papillae separate or when they form close groups produced by the mucous membranes shrinking. This always corresponds with serious health disturbance in the organism, for example in cases of internal heat or *qi* emptiness in terms of Chinese medicine.

A granular tongue with rough and swollen papillae, which can sometimes look inflamed and protruding as much as thorns do on a plant, is the result of a conversion of filiform papillae into fungiform ones. At the same time, the supply of blood to the mucous membrane vessels increases to the extent that the converted fungiform papillae are congested with blood and, therefore, look red and swollen.

A dry tongue is either the result of decreased production of saliva or the consequence of a diminished aqueous part of the saliva. This can come about when the entire organism is dehydrated or when the blood density increases, that is, with an increased hematocrit. In such cases, the secretion of saliva decreases, resulting in a dry tongue surface and in thirst. Chinese medicine maintains that a dry tongue is the most reliable clinical sign of a loss of water in the human system, since all kinds of dehydration of various origin can be easily detected by inspecting the tongue.

The term "*yin* emptiness" has its origins in the theory of traditional Chinese medicine. In such cases, the production of saliva is also decreased and as a result the surface of the tongue becomes dry. This is a condition which is also well known to Western medicine, indicating physical overexertion, a heat influence, or severe psychological strain.

According to modern Western medicine, the sympathetic tone is elevated in patients with a *yin* deficiency, whereas the parasympathetic tone is lowered. In such a state, the caliber of the blood vessels narrows as the result of an effect caused by the surrounding autonomous nerve fibers. Consequently, additional blood is forced into the tongue and causes its red discoloration. A person with such a reddened tongue may also show symptoms of high blood pressure (hypertension).

A slanting tongue deflected towards the paralyzed side signifies unilateral impairment of the hypoglossal nerve (twelfth cranial nerve), either in its central or peripheral course. This occurs in cerebral hemorrhage (stroke), brain injury, or brain tumors. The visible lesion of the motor innervation of the tongue is caused by a paralysis of the genioglossus muscle on the diseased side with a preponderance of muscle activity of the genioglossus muscle on the healthy side.

In most cases the cause of a cerebral hemorrhage resulting in a stroke is bleeding into the internal capsule where the pyramidal tract passes. The hypoglossal nerve leaves the brain via numerous roots in the area of the medulla oblongata between the pyramid and the olive (Cf. Fig **13e**, p. 39). The nerve passes through the hypoglossal canal, continues anteriorly between the internal jugular vein and the internal carotid artery, and inserts with its lingual branches above the posterior margin of the floor of the mouth into the tongue. It has close connections with the superior spinal nerves. The motor decussation of the pyramidal nerve fibers is named after the giant pyramidal cells of the precentral (motor) gyrus in the cerebral cortex and is located inferior to the exit of the hypoglossal nerve. The precentral gyrus is the principal, motor gyrus of the frontal brain lobe from where the motor fibers for the active movements of the contralateral side of the organism depart. The slanting tongue points to the paralyzed side of the body because the paralyzed genioglossus muscle is innervated by the contralateral hypoglossal nerve, which leaves the medulla oblongata superior to the pyramidal decussation.

Changes of the Coating of the Tongue

Changes in the coating of the tongue are classified according to changes in its color or its shape. From the point of view of orthodox medicine an increase in filiform papillae, especially of the callous ends at their split tips, plays a role in the appearance of the coating. In addition, changes in the moistness of the mucous membranes of the tongue and the amount of fluid available in the mouth are also considered especially important.

A yellowish coating occurs due to a further increase in the callous ends of the filiform papillae, and in such cases even a slight inflammation of the surface of the tongue can occur. A yellow discoloration can also be due to bacterial influence.

A black coating is related to a very strong increase in the callous ends of filiform papillae, giving the surface of the tongue a brownish-black appearance resulting from the massive proliferation of callous protuberances. Black discoloration can also be caused by the growth of certain types of fungi. According to modern medicine, a black coating of the tongue can be related to many different factors. These are, for example, high fever accompanied by dehydration, infectious or chronic diseases, functional disorders in the stomach and intestines, fungus infection, as well as long-term and thoughtless application of antibiotics.

If the coating thickens, the reason may be that the patient is eating very little or consuming only liquid or semi-liquid food. This decreases the mechanical friction at the surface of the tongue caused by the normal intake of food. A thick coating can also be due to high fever and following dehydration, when the production of saliva decreases. This in turn also impairs the natural cleansing mechanism of the tongue. If the filiform papillae become longer, the coating can also become thicker.

10 Summary and Outlook

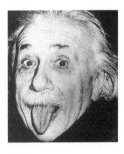

Albert Einstein, the Nobel laureate, exposes his tongue to the world. Why does he? Because the human tongue is an archetypal organ which casts a disarming spell on the observer as far as intellectual quibbels are concerned. Such a spontaneous reaction, as seen here, proves that showing one's tongue has an important function in human interaction, something which adds important elucidating information to our primarily medical context: Einstein's tongue subconsciously closes the gap between body and mind, nature and spirit, the Cartesian split between res extensa and res cogitans which is still fundamental to the natural sciences and to modern medicine. Such an emotional reaction cannot be fully explained by natural scientific thinking.

Conventional medicine is split up and separated into innumerable heterogeneous subspecialties. No physician or healer in the world of today is able to summarize, let alone control, all the manifold healing methods involved. Thus, the demonstration and evaluation of the tongue could surprisingly lead the practising doctor of our day back to his or her original task, namely to an understanding and a responsible therapy of his or her individual patient as an integrate unity.

However, there is another aspect to be considered in this context: Poor Einstein is ailing. According to Chinese diagnosis, his tongue reveals a *yin* emptiness with rising emptiness–fire. Numerous fissures and creases make the area of the middle burner look chapped. Einstein's tongue is narrow, tense, and slightly shrunken, its edges look puffy and wrinkled. As a result of his weakened *yin*, Einstein has probably suffered from insomnia. He may have been affected by a stomach disorder and constipation. The swollen edges signify a liver problem with rising liver *yang*, a condition which presumably urged him to stick his tongue out at obtrusive press people and paparazzi.

The young chimpanzee's overleaf shows no sign of a pathological development in his system.

The appropriate and effective treatment for the Nobel prize winner would have consisted of needle therapy by puncturing the foramina Spleen 6, Liver 3 and 14, Kidney 3, Bladder 15, 18, and 23, Conception Vessel (*ren mai*) 12 and Stomach 36.

He would, in addition, have benefited from herbal decoctions such as warm soups made from *Magnolia officinalis, Citrus reticulata, Glycyrrhiza uralensis, Bupleurum chinense, Scutellaria baicalensis, Pinellia ternata, Panax Ginseng, Paeonia lactiflora,* and *Ziziphus jujuba*. This could have balanced his disorder and alleviated his scorn.

Einstein's psychosociosomatic problem cannot be properly described according to standard diagnoses of conventional modern medicine. Western physicians would not even interpret his situation as a "disease" because there are no tangible pathological findings involved in the foreground. Only the amazing instrument of tongue diagnosis can show the medical reality and guide us to the right approach to an effective therapy.

NB: By comparing the two tongues it is easy to realize that our little chimpanzee feels much better and is probably happier than the famous physicist.

As pointed out above, the appropriate treatment for Einstein in his time would have consisted of acupuncture and herbal prescriptions according to a differentiating Chinese syndrome diagnosis (*bian zheng*). This treatment is not primarily geared toward a Western diagnosis applying laboratory data and radiographs, or using the reductionist terms of psychology and psychiatry such as neurosis, mental depression, psychopathy, or hysteria. Such suppositions are too inaccurate as far as the patient Einstein as an individual **being** is concerned. It follows that the actual medical reality taking the integrate unity of the person into account is beyond objective measurements, data, and reductionist terms.

The German philosopher Martin Heidegger explained the term "science" (Ger. *Wissenschaft*) in a statement as follows:

> Science in general can be defined as the totality of fundamentally coherent true propositions … within which the objectives of science are presented regarding their ground, and this means that they are understood. (From Heidegger's *Being and Time* and *Identity and Difference*, cf. *Bibliographical References*)

Now conventional Western physicians have the chance to broaden their outlook by inspecting the human tongue and by incorporating the result into their medical analysis. The outcome will be a highly personalized diagnosis which corresponds with the **individual patient as a whole**. In other words: Tongue diagnosis enables the doctor to understand his or her client in real and rationally, regarding the "**ground** (Lat. *ratio*) namely the principle of **fundamentally coherent true propositions**." And that is why such a comprehensive diagnosis can make a full claim to represent medical truth, especially when it is also underpinned by the objective findings, measurements, and data provided by the clinical experience and expertise of orthodox Western medicine. This could be the outlook towards a **New Global Medicine**: Amalgamating the Old with the New in medicine as the popular Chinese proverb "*Ku wei chin-yung*" ("Using the past for the present") suggests. Tongue diagnosis was handed down to us by ancient texts like the *Nei Jing* and other famous books from early times. But it is not at all antiquated. On the contrary. It can be linked to modern anatomy, embryology, and physiology, as well as to comprehensive clinical experience. Thus, it adds new contrast and deeper insight into Western and Eastern ways of medical therapies.

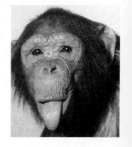

Appendix

Selected Bibliographical References

Despopoulos A, Silbernagl S. *Colour Atlas of Pathophysiology*, 5th ed. Stuttgart, New York: Georg Thieme Verlag; 2003.

Drews U, *Colour Atlas of Embryology*, Stuttgart, New York: Georg Thieme Verlag; 1995

Feneis H, *Pocket Atlas of Human Anatomy*, 4th fully rev. ed. Stuttgart, New York: Georg Thieme Verlag; 2000.

Goethe JW. *Gedenkausgabe der Werke, Briefe und Gespräche*, (Commemorative ed. of his work, letters and conversations), Zürich: Artemis, 1950.

Gray's Anatomy, 36th edition, Churchill-Livingstone, Edinburgh 1980.

Heidegger M. *Sein und Zeit* (Being and Time). 15th ed., Tübingen: Max Niemeyer Verlag, 1984, p. 11.

Heidegger M. *Being and Time, A Translation of Sein und Zeit* by Joan Stambaugh, State University of New York Press, Albany 1996.

Heidegger M. *Identität und Differenz* (Identity and Difference), Verlag Günther Neske, Pfullingen 1957, p. 78.

Huang-ti Nei-Ching Ling-Shu, Original ed. Wuhan; 1852.

Huang-ti Nei-Ching Su-Wen, Basic discourses, Part 1 of the Yellow Emperor's Classic of Internal Medicine. New ed., Beijing: Publishing House of the People's Hygiene; 1963.

Kastner J. *Chinese Nutrition Therapy*. Stuttgart, New York: Georg Thieme Verlag; 2004.

Kendall D. *DAO of Chinese Medicine, Understanding an Ancient Healing Art*, Oxford University Press, New York, Hongkong, 2002.

Mann F, *Textbook of Acupuncture*, William Heinemann Medical Books, London, 1987.

Mann F, *Reinventing Acupuncture*, A New Concept of Ancient Medicine, Butterworth Heinemann Medical Books, London, 1992

Mitchell, Feng Y, Wiseman N. *Shang Han Lun. On Cold Damage. Translation and Commentaries.* Brookline, MA: Paradigm Publications; 1990.

Needham J. *Science and Civilisation in China, Volume II*, Cambridge University Press, 1956.

Paracelsus, Theophrastus von Hohenheim. *Sämtliche Werke* (Theophrastus of Hohenheim, compl. works), St. Gallen: Facsimile reproduction, 1947

Schnorrenberger CC. *Lehrbuch der chinesischen Medizin für westliche Ärzte* (Textbook of Chinese Medicine for Western Physicians) (in German), 3rd ed., Stuttgart: Hippokrates Verlag, 1985.

Schnorrenberger CC. *Morphological Foundations of Acupuncture*: An Anatomical Nomenclature of Acupuncture Structures. In: Acupuncture in Medicine, Journal of the BMAS, November 1996, vol. XIV No 2.

Schnorrenberger CC. *Chen-Chiu – The Original Acupuncture*: A New Healing Paradigm. The Far Eastern Challenge of Needle and Moxa Therapy: Model for an Improved Medicine. Boston: Wisdom Publications, 2003.

Schnorrenberger CC. *The Anatomic and Topographic Foundations of Chinese Acupuncture and Auriculotherapy*, 6th edition (in German), published by Hippokrates Verlag, Stuttgart, 1992.

Schnorrenberger CC. *Compendium Anatomicum Acupuncturae, Textbook and Atlas of Anatomical Structures of Acupuncture* (in German), Berlin: W. De Gruyter, 1996.

Schnorrenberger B. *Abnehmen Einmal Anders* (Slimming in a Different Way), A Dietary Program According to the Five Elements, (in German) TRIAS Verlag-Georg Thieme Verlag, Stuttgart 2000.

Sun Szu-miao, *Ch'ien-chin Yi-fang (Thousand Golden Prescriptions)*, Beijing: Publishing House of the People's Hygiene, 1955

Sun Szu-Miao, *Pei-chi Ch'ien-chin Yao fang (The Valuable Thousand Golden Prescriptions)*, new ed., Shanghai: Publishing House of the People's Hygiene, 1984.

Unschuld PU, *Huang Di Nei Jing Su Wen*, University of California Press; 2003.

Wieger L. *Chinese Characters. Their origin, etymology, history, classification and signification*, Paragon Book Reprint Corp., New York; Dover Publications, Inc., New York 1965.

Wiseman N. *Glossary of Chinese Medical Terms*, Brookline, MA: Paradigm Publications; 1990.

Wiseman N., Feng Y., *A practical Dictionary of Chinese Medicine*. Brookline, MA: Paradigm Publications; 1998.

Zhang Zhong-Jing, *Shang-Han-Lun* (Treatise on Cold Diseases), Original edition, Beijing 1889.

Zhong-Yi She-Zhen (Chinese Tongue diagnosis). Ed. by the Academy of Traditional Chinese Medicine (Dept of Theoretical Foundations), Ren-Min Wei-Sheng Chu-Ban-She, Beijing 1977.

Figure Sources

Figs. 1–4: GRICMED, German Research Institute of Chinese Medicine, Freiburg: Seminar scripts. 5th ed. Freiburg 1996.

Fig. 5: Probst R, Grevers G, Iro H. *Hals-Nasen-Ohren Heilkunde*. Stuttgart, New York: Georg Thieme Verlag; 2004. [73, Fig. 4.4]

Fig. 6: Ulfig N. *Kurzlehrbuch Histologie*. Stuttgart, New York: Georg Thieme Verlag; 2003. [128, Fig. 7.5]

Fig. 7: Strutz J, Mann W. *Praxis der HNO-Heilkunde, Kopf- und Halschirurgie*. Stuttgart, New York: Georg Thieme Verlag; 2001. [98, Fig. 4.3]

Fig. 8: Barop H. *Lehrbuch und Atlas Neuraltherapie nach Huneke*. Stuttgart: Hippokrates Verlag; 1996. [161, Fig. 59]

Fig. 9: Feneis H, Dauber W. *Pocket Atlas of Human Anatomy*. Stuttgart, New York: Georg Thieme Verlag; 2000. [197, Fig. B]

Fig. 10: Rohkamm R. *Color Atlas of Neurology*. Stuttgart, New York: Georg Thieme Verlag; 2004. [21]

Fig. 11a: Strutz J, Mann W. *Praxis der HNO-Heilkunde, Kopf- und Halschirurgie*. Stuttgart, New York: Georg Thieme Verlag; 2001. [103, Fig. 4.6]

Fig. 11b: Probst R, Grevers G, Iro H. *Hals-Nasen-Ohren Heilkunde*. Stuttgart, New York: Georg Thieme Verlag; 2004. [73, Fig. 4.4]

Fig. 12: Faller A, Schuenke M. *The Human Body*. Stuttgart, New York: Georg Thieme Verlag; 2004. [591, Fig. 13.33]

Figs. 13a–e: Platzer W. *Taschenatlas der Anatomie. Band 1. Bewegungsapparat*. Stuttgart, New York: Georg Thieme Verlag; 1991.

Fig. 14: Weber T. *Memorix Zahnmedizin*. Stuttgart, New York: Georg Thieme Verlag; 2003. [189]

Fig. 15: Faller A, Schuenke M. *The Human Body*. Stuttgart, New York: Georg Thieme Verlag; 2004. [393, Fig. 9.5, after Silbernagl and Despopoulos]

Fig. 16: Drews U. *Color Atlas of Embryology*. Stuttgart, New York: Georg Thieme Verlag; 1995. [309]

Figs. 17–162: Author's drawing (Fig. 19) and photographs: Schnorrenberger C C. *Die Zungendiagnose—Zentrum der Chinesischen Medizin*. A scientific documentary. Edition Gelber Kaiser (GRICMED Publications). Freiburg: Deutsches Forschungsinstitut für chinesische Medizin; 1990.

Food Groups According to the Five Elements

Wood Nutriments

❶ Warm Food from the Wood Element

Cereals:	Meat:	Herbs/Spices:
Spelt	Chicken	Parsley
	Turkey	Vinegar (balsamic)

❷ Refreshing Food from the Wood Element

Cereals:	Fruit:	Milk products:
Durum wheat	Sour apples	Soured milk
Wheat	Berries	Buttermilk
Vegetables:	Oranges	Mozzarella cheese
Sauerkraut	Cherries	Kefir, curd cheese
Sprouts	Grapes	**Drinks:**
Pickled gherkin	**Meat:**	Fruit juices
	Duck	Rose-hip tea
		Fruit tea
		Balm-mint
		White whine
		Champagne
		Tea
		Top-fermented beer (*Weizenbier*)

❸ Cold Food from the Wood Element

Vegetables:	Fruit:	Milk products:
Sorrel	Pineapple	Yogurt
Tomatoes	Kiwi	
	Rhubarb	
	Lemon	

Fire Nutriments

❶ Hot Food from the Fire Element

Meat:
Mutton
Lamb
Sheep
Goat
All kinds of
grilled meat

Drinks:
Mulled claret
Cognac
Grog
Cordial bitters

❷ Warm Food from the Fire Element

Cereals:
Buckwheat
Milk products:
Sheep's cheese
Goat's milk
Goat's cheese

Spices:
Mugwort
Oregano
Poppy seed
Paprika
Rosemary
Thyme

Drinks:
Coffee
Cocoa
Corn coffee
Red wine
Vermouth

❸ Neutral Food from the Fire Element

Vegetables and salad
Corn salad
Brussels sprouts
Arugula

❹ Refreshing Food from the Fire Element

Cereals:
Rye
Vegetables:
Artichoke

Chicory
Green salad (lettuce)
Endive salad
Dandelion leaves

Olives
Beet
Radicchio (salad)

❺ Cold Food from the Fire Element

Drinks:
Chinese green tea
Black tea

Yarrow tea
Dandelion tea
Beer (lager)

Wormwood

Earth Nutriments

❶ Hot Food from the Earth Element

Herbs:	Drinks:	Meat:
Fennel seeds	Fennel tea	Beef broth
Cinnamon	Aniseed tea	

❷ Warm Food from the Earth Element

Cereals:	Fruit:	Pistachios
Rice	Apricot	Walnuts
Vegetables:	Peach	Sesame
Fennel	Sweet cherries	**Drinks:**
Chestnut	Raisins	Mead
Pumpkin	Mango	Liqueur
Sweet potatoes	**Nuts and Spices:**	
	Pine nuts	

❸ Neutral Food from the Earth Element

Cereals:	Vegetables:	Meat:
Millet	Cabbage	Beef
Corn	Beans	Veal
Sweeteners:	Peas	Pork
Honey	Carrots	**Milk products:**
Malt	Turnips	Eggs, butter,
Marzipan	**Fruit:**	and cream
Cane sugar	Date	Cow's milk
Drinks:	Fig	Cheese
Malt beer	Grape	**Nuts and Seeds:**
Grape juice	Plum	Peanuts
Infusion of		Hazelnuts
Glycyrrhiza		Coconut
uralensis		Almonds
		Sesame

❹ Refreshing Food from the Earth Element

Cereals:
Barley
Yeast bread
Vegetables:
Eggplant
Oyster mushrooms
Avocado
Cauliflower
Broccoli
Button mushrooms
Chinese cabbage
Cucumber
White beet (mangle)

Paprika
Comfrey
Celery
Asparagus
Spinach
Zucchini
Soy products:
Tofu
Soymilk
Fruit:
Sweet apples
Pears
Honey melon

Papaya
Herbs/Spices:
Tarragon
Nuts:
Cashew nuts
Sunflower seeds
Salad oil:
Olive oil
Sesame oil
Soy oil
Sunflower oil
Wheat germ oil
Drinks:
Apple juice
Vegetables juice

❺ Cold Food from the Earth Element

Vegetables:
Cucumber

Fruit:
Banana
Mango
Watermelon

Metal Nutriments

❶ Hot Food from the Metal Element

Herbs/Spices:
Cayenne pepper
Chilli
Curry powder
Nutmeg
Cloves
Pepper
Pimento
Aniseed
Tabasco

Drinks:
Brandy, schnapps
Whiskey
Vodka
Indian yogi tea

❷ Warm Food from the Metal Element

Cereals:
Oats

Vegetables:
Onions and
onion plants
Leek
Horseradish

Herbs/Spices:
Basil
Cumin
Dill
Ginger
Cardamom

Garlic
Coriander
Caraway seed
Lovage
Bay leaf
Marjoram
Chives
Mustard

Meat:
Pheasant
Venison
Roe deer

Wild boar

Milk products:
Harzer cheese
Munster cheese
Stilton

Drinks:
Rice wine
Sherry

❸ Refreshing Food from the Metal Element

Vegetables:
Kohlrabi
Red radish
White radish

Meat:
Goose
Turkey

Herbs/Spices:
Cress

Drinks:
Mint tea

Water Nutriments

❶ Warm Food from the Water Element

Fish:
Eel
Perch
Trout
Prawn, shrimps

Lobster
Cod
Salmon
Plaice, sole
Crayfish

Mussel
Anchovy
Tuna

❷ Neutral Food from the Water Element

Peas and beans
Adzuki beans
Peas
Lentils

Red soybean
Broad bean

❸ Refreshing Food from the Water Element

Peas and beans:	**Cereals**
Yellow and black soybeans	Wild rice
Chickpeas	

❹ Cold Food from the Water Element

Peas and beans:	**Fish:**	**Herbs/Spices:**
Mung beans	Oysters	Salt
Algae	Caviar	Soy sauce
		Drinks:
		Mineral water

Cooking Methods

Methods for Reinforcing *Yin*

- Blanching.
- Cooking with refreshing ingredients like lemon or algae.
- Freezing.
- Cooking with plenty of water.
- Cooking for a short time.

Methods for Reinforcing *Yang*

- Grilling, toasting, roasting.
- Baking.
- Smoking (e.g., ham).
- Browning.
- Pickling.
- Cooking for a long time.
- Adding warm or hot spices like chili, pepper, paprika, cloves, ginger, and cinnamon.

The Groups of Chinese Materia Medica

The 21 Classical Groups

Group 1   Remedies for opening up the surface (*jie biao yao*)

Group 1a   Pungent and warming herbs for opening up the surface (*xing wen jie biao yao*)

Group 1b   Pungent and cooling herbs for opening up the surface (*xiu liang jie biao yao*)

Group 2   Herbs for cooling heat (*qing re yao*)

Group 2a   Cooling heat and excreting fire (*qing re xie huo yao*)

Group 2b   Cooling heat and refreshing blood (*qing re liang xue yao*)

Group 2c   Cooling heat and drying wetness (*qing re zao shi yao*)

Group 2d   Cooling heat and detoxifying (*qing re jie du yao*)

Group 2e   Cooling heat and clearing the eyes (*qing re ming mu yao*)

Group 2f   Sinking emptiness heat (*tui xu re yao*)

Group 3   Dissolving phlegm, relieving cough and respiratory distress (*hua tan zhi ke ping chuan yao*)

Group 3a   Warm and dry herbs dissolving phlegm caused by cold (*wen hua han tan yao*)

Group 3b   Cooling heat and dissolving phlegm (*qing re hua tan yao*)

Group 3c   Relieving cough and respiratory distress (*zhi ke ping chuan*)

Group 4   Aromatic herbs dissolving wetness (*fang xiang hua shi yao*)

Group 5   Herbs promoting digestion (*xiao dao yao*)

Group 6   Herbs regulating qi (*xing qi yao*)

Group 7	Purgatives (*xie xia yao*)
Group 7a	Cathartics (*gong xia yao*)
Group 7b	Laxatives (*run xia yao*)
Group 7c	Strong laxatives (*run xia zhu shu yao*)
Group 8	Vermifuges (*chu chong yao*)
Group 9	Refreshing herbs restoring life and opening up blockages within the heart (*fang xiang kai qiao yao*)
Group 10	Herbs warming up the internal organs (*wen li yao*)
Group 11	Calm the liver and extinguish liver–wind (*ping gan xi feng yao*)
Group 11a	Extinguish wind and stop convulsions (*xing feng zhi jing yao*)
Group 11b	Calm the liver and suppress rising *yang* (*ping gan qian yang yao*)
Group 12	Herbs calming the mind (*an shen yao*)
Group 13	Draining water and wetness (*zhu shui shen shi yao*)
Group 13a	Excreting water, dissolving edema, opening up the urinary tract (*li shui tui zhong tong lin yao*)
Group 13b	Excreting water and treating jaundice (*li shui tui huang yao*)
Group 14	Antirheumatics expelling wind and wetness (*qu feng shi yao*)
Group 15	Hemostatic (*zhi xue yao*)
Group 16	Invigorate blood and dissolve blood blockages (*huo xue hua yu yao*)
Group 17	Cancer-controlling herbs (*zhi ai yao*)
Group 18	Pain-relieving herbs (*zhi tong yao*)

List of Chinese Materia Medica

The 21 groups of Chinese medicinal herbs, minerals, and animal products listed above not only classify the different effects of the components of a prescription but also reflect the theory of Chinese medicine. That is why every acupuncturist and Chinese doctor must be familiar with them. The erroneous assumption that Chinese medicine mainly consists of acupuncture is a grave but widespread fallacy. In a genuine Chinese treatment needles and herbs belong together and should be applied together. This has been explained in detail in the present book. Moreover, the client of Chinese medicine will highly esteem additional dietary advice from her or his doctor, as this is an essential part of traditional Chinese healing, too.

The suggestions for herbal prescriptions in Chapters 5 and 6 were compiled in accordance with the two most important historical Chinese texts on medical prescription: The *Shang Han Lun* and the *Jin Gui Yao Lüe*, both collected and created by *Zhang Zhong Jing* (AD 142–220), the famous clinician, author, and teacher of the later *Han* dynasty (AD 25–221). This unique doctor *Zhang* was sometimes (though in a defective comparison) named "the Chinese Hippocrates," which was meant to be an honorary title underlining his importance for the development of medicine. *Zhang* is the originator of the Differentiating Syndrome Diagnosis (*bian zheng*), which is, just like the whole corpus medicinae sinensis, based on the book *Huang Di Nei Jing. Zhang's* ingenious medical approach has remained valid to this day; it constitutes the highly sophisticated core of Chinese medicine as an unmatched method of healing.

Alphabetical List of the Chinese Materia Medica

A

Acacia catechu (Hua-Er-Cha) → Group XXI
Acalypha australis (Tie-Xian) → Group IId
Acanthopanax gracilistylus (Wu-Jia-Pi) → Group XIV
Achyranthes bidentata → Group XVI
Aconitum brachypodum (Xue-Shang-Yi-Zhi-Hao) → Group XVIII
Aconitum carmichaeli (Chuan-Wu) → Group XVIII
Aconitum carmichaeli (Fu-Zi) → Group X
Acorus gramineus (Shi-Chang-Pu) → Group IX
Acorus gramineus/A. calamus (Shi-Cang-Pu) → Group IV
Acronychia pedunculata (Jiang-Zhen-Xian) → Group XV
Actinidia arguta (Teng-Li-Gen) → Group XVII
Adenophora tetraphylla (Sha-Shen) → Group XIXd
Agastache Rugosa (Huo-Xian) → Group IV
Agrimonia pilosa (He-Cao-Ya) → Group VIII
Agrimonia pilosa (Xien-He-Cao) → Group XV
Akebia trifoliata (Mu-Tong) → Group XIIIa
Alangium chinense (Ba-Jiao-Feng) → Group XVIII
Alaun (Ming-Fan) → Group XXI
Albizzia julibrissin (He-Huan) → Group XII
Alisma plantago-aquatica (Ze-Xie) → Group XIIIa
Allium fistulosum L. (Cong-Bai) → Group Ia
Allium macrostemon (Xie-Bai) → Group VI
Allium sativum (Da-Suan) → Group XXI
Alpinia katsumadai Hay (Cao-Dou-Kou) → Group IV
Alpinia officiniarum (Gao-Liang-Jiang) → Group X
Alpinia oxyphylla (Yi-Zhi-Ren) → Group XX
Aluminiumsilikat (Chi-Shi-Zhi) → Group XX
Amber/Bernstein (Hu-Po) → Group XII
Amomum cardamomum (Bai-Dou-Kou) → Group IV
Amomum tsao-ko C (Cao-Guo) → Group IV
Amomum villosum (Sha-Ren) → Group IV
Andrographi paniculata (Chuan-Xin-Lian) → Group IId
Anemarrhena asphodeloides (Zhi-Mu) → Group IIa
Angelica dahurica (Bai-Zhi) → Group Ia
Angelica pubescens (Du-Huo) → Group XIV
Angelica sinensis (Dang-Gui) → Group XIXc
Apis cerana (Feng-Mi) → Group XIXa

Aquilaria agallocha (Cheng-Xiang)	→ Group VI
Araca catechu (Bing-Lang)	→ Group VIII
Arca granosa (Wa-Leng-Zi)	→ Group IIIb
Arctium lappa L. (Niu-Bang-Zi)	→ Group Ib
Ardisia crenata (Zhu-Sha-Gen)	→ Group IId
Ardisia japonica (Zi-Jin-Niu)	→ Group IIIc
Areca catechu (Da-Fu-Pi)	→ Group VI
Arisaema consanguineum (Tian-Nan-Xing)	→ Group IIIa
Aristolochia contorta (Ma-Dou-Ling)	→ Group IIIc
Aristolochia debilis (Qiang-Mu-Xiang)	→ Group XVIII
Arsenolite (Pi-Shi)	→ Group XXI
Arsensulfid (Xiong-Huang)	→ Group XXI
Artemisia apiaceae (Qing-Song)	→ Group IIf
Artemisia argyi or vulgaris (Ai-Ye)	→ Group X
Artemisia capillaris (Yin-Chen)	→ Group XIIIb
Asarum heterotropoides (Xi-Xin)	→ Group Ia
Asparagus cochinchinensis (Tian-Men-Dong)	→ Group XIXd
Aster tartaricus (Zi-Wan)	→ Group IIIc
Astragalus complanatus (Sha-Yuan-Ji-Li)	→ Group XIXb
Astragalus membranaceus (Huang-Qi)	→ Group XIXa
Atractylodes lancea (Cang-Zhu)	→ Group IV
Atractylodes macrocephala (Bai-Shu)	→ Group XIXa

B

Belamcanda chinensis (She-Gan)	→ Group IId
Benincasa hispida (Dong-Gua-Pi)	→ Group XIIIa
Berberis julianae (San-Ke-Zhen)	→ Group IIc
Bidens bipinnata (Gui-Zhen-Cao)	→ Group IId
Biota orientalis (Bai-Zi-Ren)	→ Group XII
Biota orientalis (Ce-Bai-Ye)	→ Group XV
Bletilla striata (Bai-Ji)	→ Group XV
Bombix mori (Ca-Sha)	→ Group XIV
Bombyx mori (Jiang-Chang)	→ Group XIa
Borax (Peng-Sha)	→ Group XXI
Boswellia carterii (Ru-Xiang)	→ Group XVIII
Brassica alba (Bai-Jie-Zi)	→ Group IIIa
Brucea javanica (Ya-Dan-Zi)	→ Group IId
Buddleia officinalis (Mi-Meng-Hua)	→ Group IIe
Bufo bufo (Chan-Su)	→ Group XXI
Bungarus multicinctus (Bai-Hua-She)	→ Group XIV
Bupleurum chinense (Chai-Hu)	→ Group Ib
Buthus martensi (Quan-Xie)	→ Group XIa

Caesalpinia sappan (Su-Mu) → Group XVI
Calcaria, CaO (Shi-Hui) → Group XXI
Calculus Bovis (Niu-Huang) → Group XIa
Callicarpa macrophylla (Zi-Zhu) → Group XV
Calomel (Qing-Fen) → Group XXI
Camptotheca acuminata (Xi-Shu) → Group XVII
Cannabis sativa (Huo-Ma-Ren) → Group VIIb
Capsella bursa-pastoris (Ji-Cai) → Group XV
Carpesium abrotanoides (He-Shi) → Group VIII
Carthamus tinctorius (Hong-Hua) → Group XVI
Cassia angustifolia (Fan-Xie-Ye) → Group VIIa
Cassia obtusifolia (Jue-Min-Shi) → Group IIe
Catharanthus roseus (Chang-Chun-Hua) → Group XVII
Celosia argenta (Qing-Xiang-Zhi) → Group IIe
Centella asiatica (Yi-Xue-Cao) → Group XIIIb
Centipeda minima (Shi-Hu-Sui) → Group Ia
Cephalanoplos segetum (Xiao-Ji) → Group XV
Cervus nippon (Lu-Rong → Group XIXb
Chaenomeles lagenaria (Mu-Gua) → Group XIV
Chelidonium majus (Bai-Qu-Cai) → Group IIIc
Chlorite schist. (Meng-Shi) → Group IIIb
Chrysanthemum indicum (Ye-Ju) → Group IId
Chrysanthemum morifolium (Ju-Hua) → Group Ib
Cibotium barometz (Gou-Ji) → Group XIV
Cimifuga heracleifolia (Sheng-Ma) → Group Ib
Cinnaber (Zhu-Sha) → Group XII
Cinnamomum camphora (Chang-Nao) → Group IX
Cinnamomum cassia (Gui-Pi, Rou-Gui) → Group X
Cinnamomum cassia Presl.(Gui-Zhi) → Group Ia
Cirsium japonicum (Da-Ji) → Group XV
Cistanche salsa (Rou-Cong-Rong) → Group XIXb
Citrus aurantium (Zi-Shi) → Group VI
Citrus medica, Citrus wilsonii (Xiang-Yuan) → Group VI
Citrus medica, var. sarcodactylus (Fo-Shou) → Group VI
Citrus reticulata (Ju-Pi) → Group VI
Citrus tangerina (Qing-Pi) → Group VI
Clematis chinensis (Wie ling-Xiang) → Group XIV
Cnidium monnieri (She-Chuang-Zi) → Group XXI
Codonopsis pilosula (Dang-Shen) → Group XIXa
Coix lachrymajobi (Yi-Yi-Ren) → Group XIIIa
Commelina communis (Ya-Zhi-Cao → Group IIa
Commiphora myrrha (Mo-Yao) → Group XVIII

Coptis chinensis (Huang-Lian) → Group IIc
Cornus officinalis (Shan-Zhu-Yu) → Group XX
Corydalis yanhusuo (Yan-Hu-Suo) → Group XVIII
Crataegus cuneata (Shan-Zha) → Group V
Croton tiglium (Ba-Dou) → Group VIIc
Cryptotympana atrata (Chan-Tui) → Group Ib
Cryptotympana atrata (Chan-Tui) → Group XIa
Cucurbita moschata (Nan-Gua-Zi) → Group VIII
Curculigo orchioides (Xiang-Mao) → Group XIXb
Curcuma aromatica (Yu-Jin) → Group XVI
Curcuma longa (Jiang-Huang) → Group XVI
Curcuma zedoaria (E-Shui) → Group XVI
Cuscuta chinensis (Tu-Si-Zi) → Group XIXb
Cymbopogon distans (Yun-Xiang-Cao) → Group Ia
Cynanchum atratum (Bai-Wei) → Group IIf
Cynanchum auriculatum (Ge-Shan-Xiao) → Group V
Cynanchum stauntoni (Bai-Qian) → Group IIIc
Cynomorium coccineum (Suo-Yang) → Group XIXb
Cyperus rotundus (Xiang-Fu) → Group VI
Cyrtomium fortunei (Guan-Zhong) → Group IId

D

Daemonorops draco (Xue-Jie) → Group XXI
Daphne genkwa (Yuan-Hua) → Group VIIc
Datura metel (Man-Tuo-Luo) → Group XVIII
Dendrobium nobile (Shi-Hu) → Group XIXd
Descurainia sophia/Lepidium apetalum (Ting-Li-Zi) → Group IIIc
Dianthus superbus (Qu-Mai) → Group XIIIa
Dichroa febrifuga (Chang-Shan) → Group IId
Dioscorea batatas (Shan-Yao) → Group XIXa
Dioscorea bulbifera (Huang-Du) → Group XVII
Dioscorea nipponica (Chuan-Shan-Long) → Group XIV
Dioscorea officinalis (Bei-Xie) → Group XIIIa
Diospyros kaki (Shi-Di) → Group VI
Dipsacus japonicus (Xu-Duan) → Group XIV
Dolichos lablab (Bian-Dou) → Group XIXa
Drynaria fortunei (Gu-Sui-Bu) → Group XIXb
Dryobalanops aromatica (Bing-Pian) → Group IX

E

Eclipta alba (Han-Lian-Cao) → Group XIXd
Elsholtzia loesneri Hand.-Mazz.(Xiang-Ru) → Group Ia
Ephedra sinica Stapf (Ma-Huang) → Group Ia

Ephedra sinica Stapf. (Ma-Huang-Gen)	→	Group XX
Epimedium macranthum (Yin-Yang-Huo)	→	Group XIXb
Equisetum hiemale (Mu-Zei)	→	Group Ib
Equisetum hiemale (Mu-Zei)	→	Group IIe
Equus asinus (E-Jiao)	→	Group XIXc
Eriobotriya japonica (Pi-Pa-Ye)	→	Group IIIc
Eriocaulon sieboldianum (Gu-Yin-Cao)	→	Group IIe
Erodium stephanianum (Lao-Guan-Cao)	→	Group XIV
Erythrina variegata (Hai-Tong-Pi)	→	Group XIV
Eucommia ulmoides (Du-Zhong)	→	Group XIXb
Eugenia caryophyllata (Ding-Xiang)	→	Group X
Eupatorium fortunei (Pei-Lan)	→	Group IV
Euphorbia humifusa (Di-Jin-Cao)	→	Group XV
Euphorbia kansui (Gan-Sui)	→	Group VIIc
Euphoria longan (Long-Yan-Rou)	→	Group XIXc
Eupolyphaga sinensis (Zhe-Chong)	→	Group XVI
Euryale ferox (Qian-Shi)	→	Group XX
Evodia rutaecarpa (Wu-Zhu-Yu)	→	Group X

F

Fermented wheat with herbs (Liu-Qu)	→	Group V
Foeniculum vulgare (Xiao-Hui-Xiang)	→	Group X
Forsythia suspensa (Lian-Qiao)	→	Group IId
Fraxinus rhynchophylla (Qin-Pi)	→	Group IIc
Frittillaria cirrhosa (Bei-Mu)	→	Group IIIb

G

Gardenia jasminoides (Zhi-Zi)	→	Group IIa
Gastrodia elata (Tian-Ma)	→	Group XIa
Gekko gecko (Ge-Jie)	→	Group XIXb
Gentiana macrophylla (Qin-Jiao)	→	Group XIV
Gentiana scabra (Long-Dan-Cao)	→	Group IIc
Gingko bilboa (Bai-Guo-Ren)	→	Group XX
Glechoma longituba (Lian-Qian-Cao)	→	Group XVI
Glycine max. (Dan-Dou-Chi)	→	Group Ib
Glycyrrhiza uralensis (Gan-Cao)	→	Group XIXa
Grifola umbellata (Zhu-Ling)	→	Group XIIIa
Gryllotalpa unispina (Lou-Gu)	→	Group XIIIa
Gynura segetum (Ju-Ye San-Qi)	→	Group XV
Gypsum, Gips, Calciumsulfat (Shi-Gao)	→	Group IIa

H

Human Hair (Xue-Yu-Tan)	→	Group XV

Haliotis diversicolor (Shi-Jue-Ming)	→ Group XIb
Hedera nepalensis (Chang-Chun-Teng)	→ Group XIV
Hematite/Hämatit (Dai-Zhe-Shi)	→ Group XIb
Hemsleya amabilis (Xue-Dan)	→ Group IId
Hordeum vulgare, Gerste (Mai-Ya)	→ Group V
Hounttuynia cordata (Yu-Xing-Cao)	→ Group IId
Hydnocarpus anthelmintica (Da-Feng-Zi)	→ Group XXI
Hypericum japonicum (Di-Er-Cao)	→ Group XIIIb
Hyriopsis cumingii (Zheng-Zhu-Mu)	→ Group XIb

I

Ilex chinensis (Si-Ji-Qing)	→ Group IId
Ilex pubescens (Mao-Dong-Qing)	→ Group XVI
Imperata cylindrica (Bai-Mao-Gen)	→ Group XV
Inula japonica (Xuan-Fu-Hua)	→ Group IIIc
Ipomoea hederacea (Qian-Niu-Zi)	→ Group VIIc
Isatis tinctoria (Ban-Lan-Gen)	→ Group IId
Isatis tinctoria (Da-Qing-Ye)	→ Group IId

J

Juglans regia (Hu-Tao-Ren)	→ Group XIXb

K

Knoxia valerianoides (Da-Ji)	→ Group VIIc
Kochia scoparia (Di-Fu-Zi)	→ Group XIIIa

L

Laminaria japonica (Kun-Bu)	→ Group IIIb
Leonurus heterophyllus (Yi-Mu-Cao)	→ Group XVI
Ligusticum sinense Oliv. (Gao-Ben)	→ Group Ia
Ligusticum wallichii (Chuan-Xiong)	→ Group XVI
Ligustrum lucidum (Nü-Zhen-Zi)	→ Group XIXd
Lilium Brownii (Bai-He)	→ Group XIXd
Lindera strychnifolia (Wu-Yao)	→ Group VI
Liquidambar orientalis (Su-He-Xiang)	→ Group IX
Litchi chinensi (Li-Zhi-He)	→ Group VI
Lithospermum erythrorrhizon (Zi-Cao)	→ Group IIb
Livistona chinensis (Kui-Shu-Zi)	→ Group XVII
Lobelia radicans (Ban-Bian-Lian)	→ Group XIIIa
Lonicera japonica (Jin-Yin-Hua)	→ Group IId
Lophaterum gracile (Dan-Zhu-Ye)	→ Group IIa
Loranthus parasiticus (Sang-Ji-Sheng)	→ Group XIV
Lycium barbarum (Gou-Qi-Zi)	→ Group XIXc

Lycium chinense (Di-Gu-Pi) → Group IIf
Lycopodium clavatum (Shen-Jin-Cao) → Group XIV
Lycopus lucidus (Ze-Lan) → Group XVI
Lygodium japonicum (Hai-Jin-Sha) → Group XIIIa
Lysmachia christinae (Jin-Qian-Cao) → Group XIIIb

M

Magnetite (Ci-Shi) → Group XIb
Magnolia liliflora (Xin-Yi) → Group Ia
Magnolia officinalis (Hou-Po) → Group VI
Mahonia bealei (Shi-Da-Gong-Lao) → Group IIc
Manis pentadactyla (Chuan-Shan-Jia) → Group XVI
Melia azedarach (Ku-Lian-Pi) → Group VIII
Melia toosendan (Chuan-Lian-Zi) → Group XVIII
Mentha arvensis L.(Bo-He) → Group Ib
Mercuric sulphide HgS (Shui-Yin) → Group XXI
Meretrix meretrix (Hai-Ge-Ke) → Group IIIb
Millettia reticulata (Ji-Xue-Teng) → Group XVI
Mirabilitum depuratum/sodium sulphate (or sulfate)
(Mang-Xiao) → Group VIIa
Morinda officinalis (Ba-Ji-Tian) → Group XIXb
Morus alba (Sang-Bai-Pi) → Group IIIc
Morus alba (Sang-Shen) → Group XIXc
Morus alba (Sang-Zhi) → Group XIV
Morus alba L. (Sang-Ye) → Group Ib
Moschus moschiferus (She-Xiang) → Group IX
Mylabris phalerata (Ban-Mao) → Group XXI
Myristica fragrans (Rou-Dou-Kou) → Group XX

N

Nelumbo nucifera (He-Ye) → Group IIa
Nelumbo nucifera (Lian-Zi) → Group XX
Nelumbo nucifera (Qu-Jie) → Group XV
Notopterygium incisium (Qiang-Huo) → Group Ia

O

Oldenlandia diffusa (Bai-Hua-She-She-Cao) → Group XVII
Omphalia lapialia (Lei-Wan) → Group VIII
Ophicalcite (Hue-Rui-Shi) → Group XV
Ophiopogon japonicus (Mai-Men-Dong) → Group XIXd
Oryza sativa (Nuo-Dao-Gen-Xu) → Group XX
Oryza sativa, Reis (Gu-Ya) → Group V
Ostrea gigas (Mu-Li) → Group XIb

P

Paederia scandens (Ji-Shi-Teng)	→	Group V
Paeonia lactiflora (Bai-Shao)	→	Group XIb
Paeonia suffructicosa (Mu-Dan-Pi)	→	Group IIb
Paeonia veitchii (Chi-Shao)	→	Group IIb
Panax ginseng (Ren-Shen)	→	Group XIXa
Panax pseudo-ginseng (San-Qi)	→	Group XV
Papaver somniferum (Ying-Su-Ke)	→	Group XX
Paratenodera sinensis (Sang-Piao-Xiao)	→	Group XX
Paris polyphylla (Zao-Xiu)	→	Group IId
Patrinia scabiosaefolia (Bai-Jiang)	→	Group IId
Pb³O4 (Qian-Fen)	→	Group XXI
Perilla frutescens (Su-Zi)	→	Group IIIc
Perilla frutescens (Zi-Su)	→	Group Ia
Peucedanum praeruptorum (Qian-Hu)	→	Group IIIc
Phellodendron amurense (Huang-Bo)	→	Group IIc
Pheretima asiatica (Qui-Yin)	→	Group XIa
Phragmites communis (Lu-Gen)	→	Group IIa
Phyllostachys nigra (Zhu-Ru)	→	Group IIIb
Phytolacca esculenta (Shang-Lu)	→	Group VIIc
Picrorhiza scrobhulariiflora (Hu-Huang-Lian)	→	Group IIf
Pinellia ternata (Ban-Xia)	→	Group IIIa
Placenta hominis (Zi-He-Che)	→	Group XIXb
Plantago asiatica (Che-Qian-Zi)	→	Group XIIIa
Platycodon grandiflorum (Jie-Gen)	→	Group IIIc
Polistes mandarinus (Lu-Feng-Fang)	→	Group XXI
Polygala tenuifolia (Yuan-Zhi)	→	Group XII
Polygonatum kingianum (Huang-Jing)	→	Group XIXa
Polygonatum offic. (Yu-Zhu)	→	Group XIXd
Polygonum aviculare (Bian-Xu)	→	Group XIIIa
Polygonum cuspidatum (Hu-Zhang)	→	Group XIIIb
Polygonum hydropiper (La-Liao)	→	Group IId
Polygonum multiflorum (He-Shou-Wu)	→	Group XIXc
Polygonum multiflorum (Ye-Jiao-Teng)	→	Group XII
Poria cocos (Fu-Ling)	→	Group XIIIa
Portulaca oleracea (Ma-Chi-Xian)	→	Group IId
Potentilla chinensis (Wei-Ling-Cai)	→	Group IId
Potentilla kleiniana (She-Han)	→	Group IId
Prunella vulgaris (Xia-Ku-Cao)	→	Group IIa
Prunus armeniaca (Xing-Ren)	→	Group IIIc
Prunus humilis (Yu-Li-Ren)	→	Group VIIb
Prunus mume (Wu-Mei)	→	Group XX
Prunus Persica (Tao-Ren)	→	Group XVI

Pseudostellaria heterophylla (Hai-er-Sheng)	→	Group XIXa
Psoralea corylifolia (Bu-Gu-Zhi)	→	Group XIXb
Pteris multifida (Feng-Wie-Cao)	→	Group IId
Pueraria lobata (Ge-Gen)	→	Group Ib
Pulsatilla chinensis (Bai-Tou-Wenig)	→	Group IId
Pycnostelma paniculatum (Xu-Chang-Qing)	→	Group XVIII
Pyrite (Zi-Ran-Tong)	→	Group XVI
Pyrola rotundifolia (Lu-Han-Cao)	→	Group XIXb
Pyrrosia sheareri (Shi-Wie)	→	Group XIIIa

Q

Quisqualis indica (Shi-Jun-Zi)	→	Group VIII

R

Raphanus sativus (Lai-Fu-Zi)	→	Group IIIa
Rhemannia fermentata (Shu-Di)	→	Group XIXc
Rhemannia glutinosa (Sheng-Di-Huang)	→	Group IIb
Rheum palmatum L. (Da-Huang)	→	Group VIIa
Rhododenron dauricum (Man-Shan-Hong)	→	Group IIIc
Rorippa montana (Han-Ca)	→	Group IIIc
Rosa laevigata (Jin-Ying-Zi)	→	Group XX
Rubia cordifolia (Qian-Cao-Gen)	→	Group XV
Rumex japonicus (Yang-Ti)	→	Group XXI

S

Saiga tartarica (Ling-Yang-Jiao)	→	Group XIa
Salvia miltiorrhiza (Dan-Shen)	→	Group XVI
Sanguisorba officinalis (Di-Yu)	→	Group XV
Saposhnikovia divariata (Fang-Feng)	→	Group Ia
Sarcandra glabra (Jiu-Jie-Cha)	→	Group XIV
Sargassum pallidum (Hai-Zao)	→	Group IIIb
Sargentodoxa cuneata (Hong-Teng)	→	Group IId
Saururus chinensis (San-Bai-Cao)	→	Group XIIIa
Saussurea lappa (Mu-Xiang)	→	Group VI
Schizandra chinensis (Wu-Wei-Zi)	→	Group XX
Schizonepeta tenuifolia (Jing-Jie)	→	Group Ia
Scolopendra morsitans (Wu-Gong)	→	Group XIa
Scrophularia ningpoensis (Xuan-Shen)	→	Group IIb
Scutellaria baicalensis (Huang-Qin)	→	Group IIc
Scutellaria barbata (Ban-Zhi-Lian)	→	Group XVII
Semiaquilegia adoxoides (Tian-Kui)	→	Group XVII
Senecio scandens (Qian-Li-Guang)	→	Group IId
Sepiella maindroni (Wu-Zei-Gu)	→	Group XX

Siegesbeckia orientalis (Xi-Xian-Cao)	→ Group XIV
Smilax glabra (Tu-Fu-Ling)	→ Group IId
Solanum lyratum (Bai-Yin)	→ Group XVII
Solanum nigrum (Long-Kui)	→ Group XVII
Sophora flavescens (Ku-Shen)	→ Group IIc
Sophora japonica (Huai-Hua)	→ Group XV
Sophora subprostrata (Shan-Dou-Gen)	→ Group IId
Sparganium stoloniferum (San-Leng)	→ Group XVI
Spirodela polyrrhiza (Fu-Ping)	→ Group Ib
Stegodon orientalis (Long-Gu)	→ Group XIb
Stellaria gypsophiloides (Yin-Chai-Hu)	→ Group IIf
Stemona japonica (Bai-Bu)	→ Group IIIc
Stenoloma chusanum (Wu-Jiu)	→ Group IId
Stephania sinica (Shan-Wu-Gui)	→ Group XVIII
Stephania tetrandra (Fang-Ji)	→ Group XIV
Strychnos pierriana (Ma-Qian-Zi)	→ Group XXI
Sulfur (Liu-Huang)	→ Group XXI

T

Talcum/magnesium silicate (Hua-Shi)	→ Group XIIIa
Terminalia chebula (He-Zi)	→ Group XX
Thalictrum ramosum (Tang-Song-Cao)	→ Group IIc
Tinospora sagitta (Jin-Guo-Lan)	→ Group IId
Torreya grandis (Fei-Zi)	→ Group VIII
Trachycarpus fortunei (Zhong-Lü-Tan)	→ Group XV
Tribulus terrestris (Bai-Ji-Li)	→ Group XIb
Trichosanthes kirilowii (Gua-Lou)	→ Group IIIb
Trichosanthes kirilowii (Tian-Hua-Fen)	→ Group IIa
Trigonella foenum-graecum (Hu-Lu-Ba)	→ Group XIXb
Triticum aestivum (Fu-Xiao-Mai)	→ Group XX
Trogopterus xanthipes (Wu-Ling-Zhi)	→ Group XVIII
Tussilago farfara (Kuan-Dong-Hua)	→ Group IIIc
Typha angustifolia (Pu-Huang)	→ Group XV
Typhonium giganteum (Bai-Fu-Zhi)	→ Group IIIa

U

Uncaria rhynchophylla (Gou-Teng)	→ Group XIa

V

Vaccaria pyramidata (Wang-Bu-Liu-Xing)	→ Group XVI
Verbena officinalis (Ma-Bian-Cao)	→ Group XVI
Viola yedoensis (Zi-Hua-Di-Ding)	→ Group IId
Vitex rotundifolia (Man-Jing-Zi)	→ Group Ib

Index